ROUTLEDGE LIBRARY EDITIONS: MARRIAGE

Volume 1

MARITAL VIOLENCE

MARITAL VIOLENCE

The Community Response

MARGARET BORKOWSKI,
MERVYN MURCH
AND
VAL WALKER

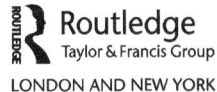

LONDON AND NEW YORK

First published in 1983 by Tavistock Publications Ltd

This edition first published in 2023
by Routledge
4 Park Square, Milton Park, Abingdon, Oxon OX14 4RN

and by Routledge
605 Third Avenue, New York, NY 10158

Routledge is an imprint of the Taylor & Francis Group, an informa business

© 1983 Margaret Borkowski, Mervyn Murch, Val Walker

All rights reserved. No part of this book may be reprinted or reproduced or utilised in any form or by any electronic, mechanical, or other means, now known or hereafter invented, including photocopying and recording, or in any information storage or retrieval system, without permission in writing from the publishers.

Trademark notice: Product or corporate names may be trademarks or registered trademarks, and are used only for identification and explanation without intent to infringe.

British Library Cataloguing in Publication Data
A catalogue record for this book is available from the British Library

ISBN: 978-1-032-46071-0 (Set)
ISBN: 978-1-032-46895-2 (Volume 1) (hbk)
ISBN: 978-1-032-46901-0 (Volume 1) (pbk)
ISBN: 978-1-003-38368-0 (Volume 1) (ebk)

DOI: 10.4324/9781003383680

Publisher's Note
The publisher has gone to great lengths to ensure the quality of this reprint but points out that some imperfections in the original copies may be apparent.

Disclaimer
The publisher has made every effort to trace copyright holders and would welcome correspondence from those they have been unable to trace.

MARITAL VIOLENCE
—the community response—

Margaret   Mervyn   Val
Borkowski   Murch   Walker

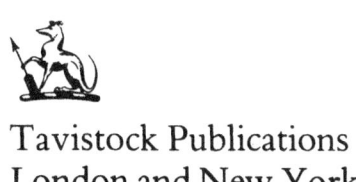

Tavistock Publications
London and New York

First published in 1983 by
Tavistock Publications Ltd
11 New Fetter Lane, London EC4P 4EE

Published in the USA by
Tavistock Publications
in association with Methuen, Inc.
733 Third Avenue, New York, NY 10017

© 1983 Margaret Borkowski, Mervyn Murch, Val Walker

Reproduced, printed and bound in Great Britain by Hazell
Watson & Viney Ltd, Aylesbury, Bucks

All rights reserved. No part of this book may be reprinted or
reproduced or utilized in any form or by any electronic,
mechanical or other means, now known or hereafter invented,
including photocopying and recording, or in any information
storage or retrieval system, without permission in writing from
the publishers.

British Library Cataloguing in Publication Data
Borkowski, Margaret
   Marital violence.
   1. Wife battering—Great Britain
   2. Legal cruelty—Great Britain
   I. Title   II. Murch, Mervyn
   III. Walker, Val
   362.8´3   HV6626

ISBN 0-422-78120-7
ISBN 0-422-78130-4 Pbk

Library of Congress Cataloging in Publication Data
Borkowski, Margaret.
   Marital violence.

   Includes bibliographical references and indexes.
   1. Wife abuse—Great Britain. 2. Family violence—
Great Britain. 3. Abused wives—Services for—Great
Britain. 4. Family policy—Great Britain. I. Murch,
Mervyn. II. Walker, Val. III. Title.
HV6626.B67   1983   362.8´3   82-19332

Contents

Acknowledgements	ix
PART I	
1 Introduction	3
2 How much marital violence comes to the attention of public services?	11
3 Some social characteristics of victims of marital violence	30
PART II	
4 Problems of definition	41
5 Problems of explanation	52
6 Questions of evidence	81
7 Issues of privacy and confidentiality	97
8 Ambivalence in victims and practitioners	115
9 Ignorance of the law is no excuse	126
10 Role definition	135
11 Perceptions of other services	167
PART III	
12 The significance of agency choice	183
13 Some policy considerations	199
Appendix The Practitioner Study: mode of sampling and characteristics of practitioners	208
References	216
Name index	223
Subject Index	226

For Adam, Giles, and Susie

Acknowledgements

Some of the ideas for the research upon which this book is based were brought to my attention by my former colleagues, Elizabeth Elston and Jane Fuller, while the three of us were investigating the circumstances of families in divorce proceedings. My first debt is therefore to them. Later, my co-authors and I refined these ideas after consulting a number of women in a West Country refuge. I am most grateful to them. I hope that the research will lead to improvement in services that will spare others some of the difficulties they had to face.

The Department of Health and Social Security commissioned and funded the research and I have welcomed close liaison with their staff, particularly Ken Corcoran and Phoebe Hall for their friendly advice, interest, and help at critical stages in the work. My thanks also to Robin Guthrie for his support while he was at the DHSS. His interest continued when he moved to the Joseph Rowntree Memorial Trust. Financial support from the Trust has enabled us to convert our original research report for the DHSS into this book.

I am also indebted to all those representatives from the legal, medical, and social services with whom we collaborated, and who arranged access to data for us. I cannot thank enough the many busy practitioners, too numerous to name, who agreed to be interviewed about their work, completed questionnaires, and taught us so much.

We benefited greatly from the expert advice of a Project Advisory Committee, the membership of which comprised Miki David, Paddy Hillyard, Annette Holman, Hilary Land, Michael Power, all from the School of Applied Social Studies at the University of Bristol; Sue Kriefman, formerly of the Department of Social Administration, University of Bristol; Daphne Norbury, British Agencies for Adoption and Fostering; Douglas Hooper, Professor of Social Work, University of Hull; and Graham Woods of the DHSS. My thanks to them all.

Throughout the project I have valued the constant but unobtrusive support and encouragement of Roy Parker, Professor of Social Administration at the University of Bristol and formerly Head of my Department, who was also Chairman of the Project Advisory Committee. Others who have contributed to the enterprise include our colleagues Kay Bader, Gwynn Davis, and Alison Macleod, and Andrew Borkowski of the Faculty of Law. I should also acknowledge the expert help of Steve Kelly from the University Computer Centre.

My thanks to Hyacinthe Harford who read the initial drafts and made many useful suggestions. Lyn Mostyn generously spent many hours reading the typescript and was of great help in our efforts to convert a research report into a book. Pat Lees typed the book with patience and meticulous care. She also compiled the index. I cannot praise her too highly.

Margaret Borkowski was the project's linchpin from beginning to end. Without her, little could have been accomplished. Val Walker was a constant source of inspiration and a skilful interviewer. She prepared the statistical data with great care. Above all, she maintained commitment to the work after she left the project and throughout a painful illness. To our distress she did not live to see the book completed.

Whatever errors and deficiencies the book may still contain are my responsibility as Project Director, and should not be held against my colleagues, advisers, and critics.

Bristol, June 1982   MERVYN MURCH

PART I

In this Part we outline the context of the research upon which this book is based, consider some of the problems associated with the collection of information on the subject, and report our findings concerning the amount of marital violence coming to the attention of public services. We also report data concerning some social characteristics of victims of marital violence obtained from several small samples of clients using public services.

1
Introduction

This book has been written for those in the legal, health, and social services from whom help is sought by people experiencing marital violence. It is based upon the findings of an investigation entitled 'The Community Response to Marital Violence'. This sought to explore the attitudes of solicitors, local authority social workers, health visitors, and general medical practitioners to marital violence. It also examined policy issues. It was commissioned by the Department of Health and Social Security and undertaken in the School of Applied Social Studies at the University of Bristol between 1977 and 1980.

Background

Some people take marital violence for granted and think that little can be done about it. For example, Mr Alex Lyon, then Minister of State at the Home Office, was reported in *The Times* (12 June 1975) to have told the Parliamentary Select Committee on Violence in Marriage that it would be 'wasting its time if it hoped to solve the difficulties of battered wives'. He added: 'In the fifteen years that I practised in the divorce court I have seen hundreds of these cases. It has been going on for years and years.'

Historically, Mr Lyon was correct. Yet marital violence is a feature of family life to which society has usually turned a blind eye. May (1978) has pointed out that 'the intermittent nature of public concern is the most striking historical feature of the problem'. Only twice in the last century has marital violence been forced into public consciousness. In the 1870s, Frances Power Cobbe's famous paper, 'Wife Torture in England' (1878), focused attention on the brutality in the 'kicking' district in Liverpool, with its annual toll of working-class women maimed or kicked to death by their husbands. Her campaign led to the Matrimonial Causes Act 1878. This gave married women the right to a legal separation and maintenance, but only after their husband had been convicted of aggravated assault. Thereafter, marital violence against women was again largely ignored by the public until

Erin Pizzey established the Chiswick Women's Aid refuge and published her book *Scream Quietly or the Neighbours Will Hear* (1971). This publication influenced the setting up of the Parliamentary Select Committee on Violence in Marriage in 1974. Nevertheless, it would probably not have been established had there not been persistent pressure from a growing feminist movement that saw marital violence as symptomatic of the more general oppression of women in a patriarchal society.

In the early 1970s the Women's Aid Federation began establishing a network of refuges. Women flocked to them, indicating something of the extent of the unmet need. By their very existence, refuges made the problem of marital violence more visible to the public. At that time, too, divorce courts provided a public arena in which some of the dimensions of the problem could be glimpsed, both in the United Kingdom (Chester and Strether 1972) and in the United States (O'Brien 1971).

Concern for marital violence was paralleled by, and to some extent associated with, a growing concern about non-accidental injury to children. This problem had received much publicity with the cases of Maria Colwell (DHSS 1974), Wayne Brewer (Somerset County Council 1977), Lisa Godfrey (London Borough of Lambeth 1975), Steven Meurs (Norfolk County Council 1975), and others, tragedies that prompted developments in social policy and social work practice. In the political campaign of 1973 which led to the setting up of the Select Committee, it was sometimes asserted that a statistical link existed between marital violence and non-accidental injury to children (Tracey 1974). Whatever the validity of this assertion, both subjects were considered by the Parliamentary Select Committee, which was later renamed the Committee on Violence in the Family. The Committee's deliberations became the political linchpin for both these matters.

The need for research

The Select Committee was unable to make any reliable estimate of the incidence of marital violence. It found that this hampered the formulation of policy, and one of its recommendations was therefore that there should be much more research. This prompted the Department of Health and Social Security, through its Homelessness and Addictions Research Liaison Group, to commission several projects,[1] the selection of which was subsequently criticized by the National

Women's Aid Federation (1981). NWAF considered that the money could have been better spent on the provision of refuges and on research undertaken by the Federation itself, since it had first-hand practical experience of the problem. Moreover, as Wilson (1976) pointed out, Government-sponsored research could be used politically to delay action:

> 'Research sometimes appears as a kind of magic solution to unpleasant problems, and a flight into research by Government and other bodies *may* be partly an attempt to shelve the problem both economically (let us not spend more money on refuges until we understand the causes for all this, then maybe we can prevent it), and emotionally (people feel something is being done and so needn't go on thinking about shocking or unpleasant problems). Also "research" somehow implies white-coated "experts" who know more about battered women than do these women themselves. And while research is very important and necessary, at the same time it is even more important and necessary to stress that there are *no* wizards and experts who have got "the answers" and that in one very real way battered women are the only experts on their own situation.' (Wilson 1976: 1)

The Bristol Project

PREVIOUS RESEARCH

Impetus for our research came from an earlier investigation of undefended divorce petitions (Elston, Fuller, and Murch 1975 and 1976) begun in 1972, after a decade in which the tide of divorce in England and Wales rose to unprecedented heights. In that study of 763 cases observed at three courts, 105 proceeded under Section 2(1) (B), the clause of the Divorce Reform Act 1969 by which divorce may be obtained on the basis of the respondent's unreasonable behaviour. In ninety-six of these cases the wife was the petitioner, and seventy women gave evidence of marital violence. Although the courts often did not require full substantiation of the facts, the details given usually indicated the frequency and severity of the violence. To illustrate this, we reproduce notes made by the researchers of five of the cases that they observed in court:

1 'Petitioner frightened by respondent's moods. Respondent had kicked her out of bed about twenty times in the last two years.

Directed by judge to relate two particular incidents, one when the respondent turned her out of the house into the rain at 1.00 a.m. and the other where he threw a bucket of cold water over her. Respondent now in mental hospital.'

2 'Order from Magistrate's Court on ground of persistent cruelty. Reconciliation after order, but respondent abused and punched petitioner afterwards. Police called in. Injunction for non-molestation granted and a ruling of "no access" to children. Respondent now in prison for contempt.'

3 'Petitioner had previously applied for injunction for non-molestation. There were a vast number of allegations: locked out after being beaten up, threats of knifing and putting petitioner "six feet under", children affected. Affidavit from doctor submitted.'

4 'History of considerable violence throughout marriage. Respondent used violence even on honeymoon. Drunk three times a week and would come back and punch petitioner. Petitioner had to go to hospital with broken jaw after respondent had punched her in the face. Petitioner had continued to live with him for the sake of the children, but in the last two years children began to be affected.'

5 'Magistrate's Court order on the grounds of adultery and persistent cruelty, but there was a reconciliation. However an injunction to restrain respondent from molesting petitioner was granted in 1972. Respondent had made petitioner "a nervous wreck". Respondent hit both petitioner and the children. Psychiatric report on the children submitted.'

When the researchers interviewed twenty-two of these women after the court hearing, it was discovered that, quite apart from the stress and suffering arising from the violence itself, many had experienced a number of problems when seeking help. The majority had initially turned to relatives and friends who, although they had provided support and sometimes temporary accommodation, often made it clear to the women that they did not want to be involved in the couple's domestic problems. Most of the women had been to their doctor, who had prescribed psychotropic drugs, invariably librium or valium. Seven said the GP had listened carefully and offered useful advice, but another seven said the GP had been unsympathetic. A few said that once they had arrived at the surgery they had felt too ashamed to talk to the doctor about the violence.

In a number of cases the police had been called. They were reported as having often taken the view that since it was a 'domestic' matter little could be done. As Jack Ashley (Hansard July 1973) said in an adjournment debate in the House of Commons, the phrase 'domestic dispute' tends to be 'parroted as an incantation for inaction'. The police told some women to contact the local authority social services. When the women did so, some mentioned that social workers had discouraged them from leaving their husband in the evident belief that they should try harder to keep the marriage together. Since there were few refuges in the early 1970s, those women who did attempt to leave had great difficulty finding accommodation where there was no risk of further assault.

Most of the women turned to solicitors after they had decided to separate. They usually wanted advice about divorce. Nineteen said that they had found the solicitor sympathetic, supportive, and a source of realistic advice. Even so, the researchers thought that in the light of the women's experiences, some of the solicitors could have done more, for example by instituting proceedings for an injunction.[2]

In the divorce court itself it was noted that court officials and judges quite often seemed curiously inured to the violence. Some officials were sceptical about women's allegations of violence, even though all the cases were undefended and the evidence was not challenged by the respondent. Later, in conversation with some practitioners, it became clear that they found it hard to believe that a woman could experience such violence and yet remain with her husband or even return to him after a short separation. Some practitioners explained this away by saying that such women came from working-class families given to rough living. Others said that the women must be neurotically punishment-seeking, or get perverse excitement from living in a violent, emotionally charged relationship. One County Court clerk said: 'What else can you believe when they tell terrible tales of brutality and then you hear that they are together again?'.

OBJECTIVES

It was against this background that we decided to investigate further the part played by services to which women had turned for help. We thought it important to explore and better understand the attitudes that women had encountered when consulting practitioners. Some practitioners were experienced as helpful, but others were seen as ambivalent, even rejecting.

While physical violence between two partners was the project's central concern, we drew its boundaries sufficiently widely to permit consideration of marital violence in the context of other overtly presented marital problems. We defined marital violence as threatened or actual physical assault by one marital partner upon the other. This definition did not attempt to introduce criteria as to the frequency of assault or the degree of injury that might have been sustained. As far as the word 'marital' was concerned, we adopted the couple's own definition of themselves as partners, whether or not they were legally married. This included those who were cohabiting as well as those who were separated or divorced but still in contact. Overall, we hoped to obtain a picture of the way services in a large city attempt to meet the needs of people with these problems.

A review of the literature and the comparatively few research findings available in 1976, and an examination of evidence to the Parliamentary Select Committee, suggested there were five key questions that agency-focused research should investigate. They provide the framework around which this book is constructed. The five questions are:

1. How much marital violence comes to the attention of public services? (Chapter 2)
2. How do practitioners working in different services view the problem of marital violence? (Chapters 4-7 and 9-11)
3. Why do women victims of marital violence often change their mind about seeking help? (Chapter 8)
4. Where do individuals with marital problems most frequently go for help and what, if any, is the significance of agency choice? (Chapter 12)
5. How effective is referral and liaison between services? (Chapters 11 and 12)

OUTLINE METHOD OF APPROACH

The research was a detailed local study, conducted in the city of Bristol, the population of which was estimated to be 578,000 in 1977. It divided into three stages:

Feasibility Study

We began the work by exploring the viability of various methods of approach. We talked with some women from a refuge, met with representatives of local services to discuss and negotiate their collaboration, and conducted a number of informal preliminary interviews with their staff in order to find out what the main difficulties would be in obtaining information.

The Agency Study

We then made a reconnaissance of those services thought likely to be approached directly by people experiencing marital violence. This meant that we did not study services that draw their clientele through intermediaries, such as specialist clinics. Nor did we examine the work of the courts, since they were not of immediate concern to our sponsors, the Department of Health and Social Security.

This part of the work had two purposes: to estimate the number of cases coming to the attention of services; and to discover what policies, if any, they employed when dealing with them. Using an open-ended checklist of questions, we interviewed members of staff at various levels of responsibility in order to obtain a reasonably representative cross-section of views. The majority of services also estimated the number of cases of marital violence coming to their attention, as will be seen in Chapter 2.

The Practitioner Study

Four occupational groups were chosen for this part of the research: doctors and lawyers because our earlier study had shown that they were most frequently used by the divorcing population; health visitors and local authority social workers because the DHSS was particularly keen that we should study their work. Each group was sufficiently large and homogeneous for individual sampling, the methodology of which is summarized in the Appendix. Information was sought in two ways: first by interview, using a structured questionnaire in which some questions were common to all while others were designed to elicit information about the individual's particular setting. Second, all practitioners were asked to complete two forms. In the first they gave details of their workload and indicated what proportion of it involved cases of known or suspected marital violence. In the second they were asked to give details of the most recent case of marital violence with which they had dealt, but not all were willing to do so. Some did not have a case they could recall sufficiently well. Others said that they were too busy to fill in the form. Nevertheless, an overall return rate of 64 per cent was achieved, providing a total of 128 cases. We have used this case material in Chapters 3 and 5.

Notes

1 Apart from our own study, research was also undertaken as part of this programme by Jan Pahl at the University of Kent and by Barbara Dawson, Tony Farragher, and Professor R. Frankenburg at the University of Keele.
2 We should point out that in 1972 there were many shortcomings in the injunction procedure, some of which have since been rectified by the Domestic Violence and Matrimonial Proceedings Act of 1976 and the Matrimonial Proceedings Magistrate's Courts Act 1978.

2
How much marital violence comes to the attention of public services?

'Once I made an appointment to see the doctor but I never kept it. I felt too embarrassed and ashamed to go really. I was badly bruised and had a cut underneath the eye. My legs were aching quite a bit – he's got a truncheon.'
(Housewife. Age: 20. Divorced. Two children in her care. Length of marriage: 3 years)

In a booklet exploring the policy issues connected with marital violence, Miller wrote, 'One fundamental issue is the estimation of the size of the demand for help – without such estimates it has proved hard to bring pressure to bear to create provision' (Miller 1975:8). In the early 1970s, wildly differing estimates about the scale of the problem were produced. For example Ashley (1973) estimated approximately 27,000 serious cases per year. Others suggested that the figure could be as high as 200,000.

The Parliamentary Select Committee on Violence in Marriage (1975) commented: 'Despite our efforts, we are unlikely to give any estimate of what the likely numbers are . . . . All witnesses are agreed on the need for research on the scale of the problem'.

Although some agencies, notably the police (see, for example, Bedfordshire Police 1976), had made small-scale studies of the number of cases of marital violence with which they had dealt in a given period, when we began our research there had been no attempt to count such incidents in other relevant services, such as general medical practice, solicitors' offices, hospital emergency departments, marriage guidance councils, and departments of social service. We decided to get some idea of the size of the problem by asking various agencies to make estimates of the number of cases of marital violence that their staff had noticed over a given period. We thought this would show whether marital violence was perceived as a numerically important problem. Nevertheless, there were formidable problems in collecting data of this kind.

Problems of data collection

Many problems arose from having to rely on other people's perception of interpersonal relations. When the subject of their concern is highly emotive and not generally well understood, as in the case of marital violence, the problems multiply. We were studying what have been termed 'surface' phenomena of perception (Heider 1958): namely what practitioners notice about their clients, what they think and feel about them, and how they think they react to them. Heider, a social psychologist, has warned that in their own way these matters are every bit as challenging and difficult to unravel and understand as less 'obvious' deeper unconscious phenomena. For example, when practitioners were telling us about cases of marital violence with which they had dealt, there was no means of verifying the facts reported to us, nor why some pieces of information had been selected as relevant and others rejected. We did not know how much original information they had available to them, and we could not tell how far that information itself had been filtered by the clients/patients themselves. In many instances, practitioners had only seen one party to the marital dispute, usually the victim, and this contributed to bias. Partners in conflict often have different views about their dispute, giving conflicting accounts to outsiders, who may be unable to get any corroborative evidence. Some victims of marital violence protect their assailants by cover-up stories, or minimize the seriousness of what happened; others exaggerate. Some practitioners will probe to test the validity of what they have been told, while others will not. Accordingly, information derived from practitioners is bound to be 'soft' and difficult to verify, and should therefore be treated with caution.

Outsiders seldom witness marital violence and have to rely on recollection. Another major problem when studying marital behaviour is how to counteract the influence of privacy so that one can get a reasonably accurate and representative picture of what happened. This creates two main difficulties when one is working through intermediaries: first, it may influence what informants tell researchers; second, it may influence what *their* informants tell them.

A further difficulty is that intermediaries inevitably view violent marriages in the light of their own professional as well as personal values and experience. This influences what they notice in the first place and what they choose to tell others. It introduces a further element of distortion. In order to contain this, one can try to structure the intermediaries' perspectives by alerting them to the kind of data required, training them to use particular definitions of marital violence, and so on. In practice, there is a limit to this. Their working experience tends to condition practitioners into the recognition and selection of the information necessary for the performance of their professional tasks.

The way practitioners define marital violence varies a good deal, as we shall see in Chapter 4. Obviously, this influences the way they report its incidence. As far as possible, we ensured that all services and practitioners who made calculations of incidents used our definition, as given in Chapter 1. We have had to assume that the information they gave us was selected on this basis. But given our findings reported in Chapter 4 about the variation in definition that practitioners themselves used, there is bound to be doubt how vigorously practitioners adopted our definition for this particular purpose.

Difficulties over the meaning of definitions are part of a wider and more fundamental problem about the use of language in quantitative research. The worst problems arise from the words people use, such as 'violence', 'force', 'conflict', 'aggression', 'anger', which can be used synonymously, but may also be given quite distinct meanings. Misunderstanding can arise even when such words are used accurately. For example, when a woman describes her husband as 'aggressive' she may only mean that he is irritable, but she could equally mean that he has a propensity for serious physical violence.

Another area of difficulty is that most practitioners and services see marital violence as a marginal issue, met with only occasionally. Apart from Women's Aid, there is no service with primary responsibility for marital violence. A practitioner may only notice signs of violence when dealing with some other presenting problem. It is hard for practitioners to generalize about a problem that they may see as marginal. Also, since they are not accustomed to dealing with it, they may fail to notice its salient features, and may either underestimate its incidence, or be so shocked that it is exaggerated and frequently recalled.

Method of approach

Given these qualifications, we set out to make a preliminary estimate of the amount of marital violence coming to the attention of various agencies working in the city of Bristol. We saw these services as collecting-points where information about the relevant clientele could be gathered. As explained in Chapter 1, we limited ourselves to those services thought most likely to be approached directly by members of the public who may experience violence in their marital relationships.

We were unable to undertake a simultaneous incident count of marital cases involving violence presenting to all the relevant agencies in the city over a given period, as we had hoped to do. The task of administering such a count would have been too complex in view of the large number of potential informants and the need to ensure that information was recorded uniformly, and the need to identify cases in order to avoid multiple presentation would have conflicted with the need to preserve confidentiality.

Findings

We report our findings in three parts:

1 From those agencies and services that agreed specifically to monitor their intake or scrutinize their total caseload.
2 From those agencies and services where estimates were made from existing agency data.
3 From doctors and solicitors where the degree of variation between practitioners rendered attempts to make generalized statements futile.

Part 1

VOLUNTARY SPECIALIST SERVICES

Avon Council on Alcoholism

The Avon Council on Alcoholism is a small, non-statutory agency which, in 1977, employed four full-time members of staff. They provide counselling and advisory services to those with a drinking problem, and help and advice to friends, relatives, and employers. During preliminary discussions, the staff told us that marital violence was a fairly familiar occurrence in problem-drinkers' lives. The counsellors agreed to monitor the agency's intake for a period of six months during 1978. The results were as follows. The overall intake was 154 cases. Six cases of marital violence were noticed, giving a ratio of one in twenty-six, or 4 per cent. About a third of the agency clientele is single (31 per cent) or widowed (5 per cent). We do not know what proportion of these would be cohabiting or regarding themselves as 'partnered' in some way.

Marriage Guidance Councils

We arranged with Bristol Marriage Guidance and the Catholic Marriage Advisory Council for new cases to be monitored for a period of six months (1 January 1977 to 30 June 1977). All counsellors working in the city agreed to help. A case-monitoring record form was designed to be completed by individual counsellors dealing with any new cases involving marital violence that they noticed.

Bristol Marriage Guidance reported ten cases in an overall intake of 289, giving a ratio of one in twenty-nine cases, or 3 per cent. The Catholic Marriage Advisory Council reported two cases in a total of forty-eight, a ratio of one in twenty-four or 4 per cent.

Before undertaking this survey Bristol Marriage Guidance estimated that one case in fifteen was thought to involve some degree of physical violence. Our survey suggests that only half that number are noticed. Unfortunately, we were unable to compare our findings with the National Marriage Guidance Council's own study of their clientele, since it produced no evidence about the prevalence of violence (Heisler and Whitehouse 1976). They classified clients' presenting problems under ten 'problem area' categories, including 'management of money', 'sexual difficulties', 'infidelity', 'personal traits', 'housing', and 'unemployment'. We can only assume that cases of marital violence, when they did occur, were classified under some of these headings, most probably 'personal traits' which comprised 55 per cent of the total.

Citizens' Advice Bureau

The Bristol Office was established in 1977, with one central office situated in the main shopping centre of the city. In order to give the agency time to establish itself it was agreed that a survey be made of agency records for new cases in the year 1 September 1978 to 31 August 1979.

The total number of cases dealt with was 28,116, of which 3,938 were classified as 'Family and Personal'. It was assumed that all cases of marital violence would be placed in this category by the CAB workers who completed the agency case-records.

Scrutiny of these 3,938 case-records revealed 105 cases in which reference was made in the agency record to marital violence.[1] This gives a ratio of one in 267. They noticed on average eleven cases of marital violence per month, the maximum number in any one month being sixteen, the minimum three.

HOSPITAL ACCIDENT DEPARTMENTS

The Bristol Royal Infirmary and Southmead Hospital are the two main general hospitals with accident departments drawing casualties from the city.[2] Following discussions with the appropriate medical authorities it was agreed that the sisters-in-charge would collect information about casualties whose injuries were believed to be caused by marital violence.

Data collection began in October 1978. The sisters-in-charge perused the medical notes of all casualties every few days, and transferred information about cases of marital violence on to specially prepared record cards. These were completed not only in cases where the patient informed medical staff that injuries were due to marital violence, but also in cases where the staff had good cause to suspect marital violence. Information was collected for sixteen months at Southmead Hospital and ten months at the BRI.[3] Table 2(1) below summarizes the findings.

Table 2(1) Cases of marital violence recorded at hospital accident departments[4]

Hospital	Nos of MV cases reported	Monthly average	Total nos of all new cases dealt with	Monthly average	Ratio of MV cases to total
Southmead (16 mths)	37	2	50,305	3144	1:1359
BRI (10 mths)	18	2	46,489	4649	1:2582

The maximum number of cases reported in any one month was six (BRI, November 1978). Both hospitals reported months when no cases were noticed at all.

Our overall impression is that cases of marital violence comprise

Marital violence and the public services 17

only a tiny proportion of the total number of accident admissions. But returns may under-represent the actual number of cases noticed. First, we had to rely on hospital staff, particularly the two sisters-in-charge, as our sole source of information. We could not check whether they always performed their task rigorously and on occasion they were working under severe pressure. On the other hand, both sisters were experienced, responsible, and keen to assist our project. Second, some patients may not have volunteered the reason for their injuries to the medical staff attending them. In any case, the staff may not always have enquired into the reasons or recorded them on the medical notes. We know of one case where a victim of marital violence went to one of the accident departments, and told the medical staff how she had sustained her injuries; this case was not recorded. This confirms our view that our system of data collection was not foolproof.

DOMICILIARY STATUTORY SOCIAL AND MEDICAL SERVICES

Health visitors

Of the fifty health visitors whom we interviewed, forty-five agreed to complete a form recording the size of their total caseload, the number of children known to them who were on the Concealed Parental Violence register, and the number of known or suspected cases of marital violence encountered during the previous twelve months. From these data we calculated that the average caseload was 312 per health visitor, the highest being 551; the lowest 125.[5]

Two-hundred-and-fifty cases of known and suspected marital violence were reported, of which 163 were classified as 'known'. A rough estimate of the average number of marital violence cases within a health visitor's caseload then emerged. The results were as follows:

a) *known* cases: 1 in 86.1 or 1.1 per cent of the caseload.
b) *known and suspected* cases: 1 in 56.2 or 1.8 per cent of the caseload.

It should be noted that these estimates assume a 'static' caseload size. In reality the total number of cases known to a health visitor over a year is likely to be a good deal higher, allowing for the in-flow of new cases and the termination of old ones. Unfortunately, we did not collect information allowing us to take these factors into consideration. Our calculations are therefore likely to overestimate the number of cases of marital violence seen in a year. This point applies equally to our data concerning local authority social workers.

Marital Violence

Local authority social workers

Thirty-six of the fifty social workers completed a form giving details of their total caseload, the number of children known to be on the CPV register, and the number of known and suspected cases of marital violence encountered during the previous twelve months. From a combined total caseload of 1,121 cases, we calculated that the average was thirty-one, the highest being forty-five, the lowest fifteen.

Social workers reported 141 known and suspected cases of marital violence of which 107 were classified as 'known'. From these data we estimate the average proportion of cases of marital violence likely to be found in a social worker's caseload to be as follows:

a) *known* cases: 1 in 10.4 or 10.5 per cent.
b) *known and suspected* cases: 1 in 7.9 or 12.5 per cent.

SUMMARY OF FINDINGS FROM PART I

Table 2(2) shows the ratio of identified cases of marital violence to total agency intake, or caseload.

Table 2(2)

	Number of cases of MV	Number of new cases
Voluntary specialist agencies:		
Avon Council on Alcoholism	1	26
Bristol Marriage Guidance	1	29
Citizens' Advice Bureau	1	267
Hospital accident departments:		
Southmead Hospital	1	1359
Bristol Royal Infirmary	1	2582
Domiciliary social and medical services:		
Health visitors	1	86.1
Local authority social workers	1	10.4

Part 2

THE POLICE

Our police data were provided by the Statistics Officer of the Avon and Somerset Constabulary and the eight Divisional Commanders responsible for policing the City of Bristol (usually Superintendent or Chief Inspector). Each had seen an outline of our research proposal. The Superintendent in Charge of Research, who arranged introductions, had asked Commanders to provide us with as much hard evidence of marital violence as was readily available. At the time of our interviews the police did not keep special records of incidents of marital violence to which they were called. Nevertheless, six of the eight Commanders made a special short-term enquiry on our behalf. The Statistics Officer provided us with details of prosecutions arising from marital violence in the city during 1977. We have therefore been able to make certain comparisons between the two sets of data, which are presented in *Table 2(3)*.

Various points emerge from these data. First, the amount of marital violence coming to police notice varies area by area. For example, the Central area, with a low residential population but containing many cinemas, night clubs, and shops, produced only one domestic violence prosecution, but the highest number of prosecutions for offences against the person. In Lockleaze, largely an area of pre-war private housing, a low incidence of domestic calls was matched by generally low prosecution figures. By contrast, 'B' Division, which covers a large area of post-war local authority housing, produced the highest incidence of both estimated domestic incidents and prosecutions for marital violence. The two sub-divisional police stations in that division were at Bishopsworth and Broadbury Road. The Southmead station to the north of the city also serves a large council housing area and the seaport of Avonmouth. In this part of the Division the incidence was about average.

Most of the Commanders interviewed had the impression that certain localities produced proportionately more 'domestic calls' than others, mentioning in this respect the larger working-class council housing estates to the north and south of the city. Some also mentioned the central 'bed-sitter' areas of Clifton, Cotham, and Redland in 'C' Division. Unfortunately, our data for these particular areas are incomplete, but on the basis of prosecution figures the incidence seems low.

More detailed analysis would be needed to establish whether or not there was a relationship between localities and incidence of marital violence. Our information suggests that such an investigation, perhaps carried out by the police themselves, would be worth while.

The low number of prosecutions in relation to the estimated

Table 2(3) *Police divisional statistics*

(a) Area	(b) Estimated resident population	(c) Estimated annual domestic incidents	(d) Ratio to population	(e) % of (c) to (b)	(f) Total all recorded Offences Against the Person 1977	(g) No. of domestic violence prosecutions 1977	(h) Ratio of 'domestic' to 'all' Offences Against the Person	(i) % of actual prosecutions (h) to estimated annual domestic incidents (c)
A Division Central	8,500	Not known	—	—	194	1	1:194	—
A Division Trinity Road	20,000	156	1:128	0.7	89	5	1:18	3.2
B Division Bishopsworth	100,000	960	1:104	0.9	66	9	1:7	0.9
B Division Broadbury Road	108,000	960	1:112	0.8	141	29	1:5	3.0
C Division Redland	65,000	Not known	—	—	75	3	1:25	—
C Division Southmead	150,000	960	1:156	0.6	77	7	1:11	0.7
D Division Lockleaze	70,000	300	1:233	0.4	94	5	1:19	1.6
D Division St George	57,000	960	1:59	1.6	45	3	1:15	0.3
Total	578,000	4,296 (for 6 areas only)	—	—	781	62	1:12	—

numbers of reported domestic incidents is striking. These results are lower than all the estimates given by the Divisional Commanders when we interviewed them during the Agency study. For example, one Commander suggested that formal charges were brought in 20 per cent of the cases brought to notice in his area, while others suggested it to be as low as 5 per cent. Yet if one looks at the data in column (i) in Table 2(3), one sees that the highest figure produced by our calculations was 3.2 per cent (Trinity Road).

Commanders gave various reasons for the small proportion of cases leading to prosecution: insufficient evidence, reluctance of wives to make formal statements against their husbands, etc. The general prosecution policy is based on the fact that individual constables dealing with complaints have wide discretion.[6] In general, the police treat minor complaints with caution and rarely institute proceedings for breach of the peace or common assault (Section 42, Offences Against the Person Act 1861). If, on the other hand, there is clear evidence of injury, a charge under Section 47 (actual bodily harm), or Section 20 (unlawful wounding), or Section 18 (grievous bodily harm) will result. The great majority of prosecutions are brought under Section 47.

Dealing with marital violence forms only a small proportion of police work. We estimate that in 1977 in Bristol the police probably attended 5,000–6,000 domestic calls, many of which they would have regarded as trivial. The total number of prosecutions that year involving marital violence under the Offences Against the Person Act 1861 was only sixty-two.

In 1975 the Avon and Somerset Constabulary published a report analysing police activity in two Divisions in the City (St George and Lockleaze) (Arkell 1975). This classified the various tasks that police officers perform. Attending 'domestic' incidents was listed under the heading 'Response to the public' together with such other activities as attending fires, investigating reports about missing persons, sudden deaths, alarms, etc. 'Domestics' comprised only 7 per cent of the time taken up by officers under this overall heading.

Unless the police make it a standard practice to record all domestic incidents to which they are called that involve possible marital violence, there will be no precise way of recording their incidence. Nevertheless, in relation to other calls on police services, the amount of work generated by marital violence seems to be marginal. By saying this we do not imply that the police do not regard it seriously. As far as the evidence received from the Divisional Commanders is

Marital Violence

concerned, it is clear that they do. As one said: 'We look upon every domestic call as a possible murder'.

BRISTOL WOMEN'S AID

This organization runs several refuges in the city for victims of marital violence and their children. It also provides general advice and information for women seeking refuge away from Bristol. The organizers kindly supplied us with the following information for the year 1977:

a) *Requests for refuge*

Number of Bristol resident women requesting refuge	88
Number of women from elsewhere requesting refuge	31
	119

These 119 women also sought shelter for 155 dependent children.

b) *Women referred to Bristol refuges: n = 77 women and 93 children*

(i) *Source of referral*

	%
Social services department	34
Self	18
Other women's aid refuge	13
Samaritans	5
Police	4
Health visitor	4
Other (solicitor, doctor, etc.)	22
	100

(ii) *Length of woman's stay*

	%
Under 1 week	39
1–4 weeks	25
1–3 months	24
Over 3 months	12
	100

(iii) *Woman's home area* %
Bristol 59
Rest of Avon 7
Other South-West towns 7
South Wales 12
Rest of UK 11
Not recorded 4
                                                                         ___
                                                                         100

c) *Women referred out of Bristol without entering Bristol refuge:*
   n = 42 women and 62 children %
   Destination:
   Other Avon refuges 47
   Other South Western refuges 26
   South Wales refuges 9
   Refuges in rest of UK 18
                                                                         ___
                                                                         100

Part 3

GENERAL MEDICAL PRACTITIONERS

The fifty doctors interviewed had insufficient time to search their records for data about patients who had presented with problems of marital violence. However, most were prepared to make rough estimates. They also told us the approximate size of their list.

Forty-six of the fifty doctors completed a form from which we gathered the following information: the average list size was 3,143 patients, compared with 2,637 for doctors working in urban areas given in the National Morbidity Survey 1971/72 (DHSS 1979: Table 5(3)). The smallest list in our survey was 1,866, and the largest 3,500. Doctors' estimates of cases of marital violence varied widely as can be seen in *Table 2(4)*.

These figures may be too vague to be of much use, since they may reflect genuine variations in the kinds of problems that patients present, possibly due to social conditions in the locality, and its demographic composition. Nevertheless, we find it interesting that

Table 2(4) GPs' estimates of frequency of meeting cases of marital violence (n = 46 doctors)

	Female victims		Male victims	
	n	%	n	%
Once a week	1	2	–	–
Once a fortnight	4	9	–	–
Once a month	16	35	1	
Once every three months	11	24	3	26
Once every six months	7	15	8	
Once a year	5	11	4	9
Less often	2	4	15	32.5
Never	–	–	15	32.5

26 per cent of the doctors considered that they encountered a male victim at least every six months despite the fact that consultation rates are almost twice as high for women as for men in the age range fifteen to forty-four (DHSS 1979: Table 9(a)).

Overall, our figures suggest that given the large number of patients that doctors see, cases of marital violence are encountered relatively infrequently, a point made by many doctors we approached, and validated by data published in the National Morbidity Survey. This survey gives statistical information about the rates of diagnosed conditions and diseases, by sex and age of patients. Most cases of marital violence would be classified under the heading 'Accidents, poisonings, and violence' in *Table 9(a)* of that report (DHSS 1979), which is transposed here in *Table 2(5)*. It should be noted that *Table 2:12* of the National Morbidity Survey shows that women in the fifteen to forty-four age range make on average 3.8 visits a year to a doctor while men of that age range make on average 2.0 visits, broadly equivalent to findings in the General Household Survey 1972 (HMSO 1975).

Cases of marital violence are only likely to make up a small proportion of the 'accident, poisonings, and violence' group. In the case of women patients, marital violence as the classified reason for consultation will be found amongst the 8 per cent of all women aged between twenty-five and forty-four who consult their doctors in any one year because of an 'accident, poisoning, or as a result of injury caused by violence'. The proportion must therefore be small and provides support for the estimates given by the doctors in our sample.

Table 2(5) *One-year patient consulting rates: percentage population at risk × sex, age, and disease grouping*

Disease or condition	Age	
	15–24 %	25–44 %
All diseases and conditions	M: 59	M: 57
	F: 76	F: 73
Accidents, poisonings and violence	M: 15.0	M: 10.7
(nature of injury)	F: 8.7	F: 7.5
Examples of other classifications for comparison:		
Diseases of the respiratory system	M: 23.9	M: 21.7
	F: 28.2	F: 25.6
Diseases of digestive system	M: 6.7	M: 7.9
	F: 8.7	F: 7.9
Diseases of the genito-urinary system	M: 1.6	M: 1.8
	F: 21.5	F: 20.5
Mental disorders	M: 5.8	M: 9.1
	F: 14.2	F: 20.6

From: Table 9(a), Studies on Medical and Population Subject Report No. 36, National Morbidity Survey.

SOLICITORS

Solicitors offer the public various services. Some deal with a whole range of legal matters, others specialize. There is little point, therefore, in trying to estimate the average size of a solicitor's caseload devoted to matrimonial work. Nevertheless, we were concerned to find out which of the fifty solicitors interviewed did most of this work, and what range of experience they had in dealing with marital violence.

Twenty-four solicitors completed a form recording the number of matrimonial cases dealt with during the previous year in the magistrate's court and the divorce court; how many of the divorce cases proceeded under Section 1(2)b of the Matrimonial Causes Act 1973 (unreasonable behaviour), a high proportion of which would rely on evidence of physical violence; and how many injunctions were granted as a result of marital violence. The one with the most cases dealt with sixty-five in the magistrate's court and 250 in the divorce court, of which eighty were 1(2)b cases. He also prepared fifteen cases which led to the grant of injunctions. The one with the least dealt with only two in the magistrate's court and eighteen in the divorce court, of which nine were 1(2)b cases and prepared four cases in which injunctions were granted.

The twenty-four solicitors from whom we received information dealt with 1,207 divorces and prepared eighty-five applications for injunctions – an average ratio of one injunction application to every fourteen divorces. Eight solicitors dealt with more than fifty divorce cases a year each, and calculations for them suggest that the proportion of the grant of injunctions to divorces is lower than our average, approximately one injunction granted to seventeen divorces. One solicitor had an injunction/divorce ratio of 1:4.5; at the other extreme one of the busiest divorce lawyers, who dealt with ninety-two divorces, only prepared four applications for injunctions, giving a ratio of 1:23. Our data suggest that the greater the volume of matrimonial work undertaken by a lawyer, the smaller the proportion of cases involving injunctions. We have not been able to examine the variables that may contribute to this proposition.

Discussion

The number of cases of marital violence coming to the notice of services may only be a small fraction of those occurring. This is suggested by recent findings obtained from the Bristol Special Procedure in Divorce project.[7] In a sample of recently divorced people, 40 per cent of 161 men interviewed and 40 per cent of the 237 women reported some physical violence in their previous marriage. This study, as yet unpublished, shows that 20 per cent of the women petitioners used evidence of their husband's violence to support a petition based on unreasonable behaviour in undefended cases. A further 20 per cent claimed that there had been episodes of physical violence, although they had chosen to base their petitions on some other evidence. This second group was rather more middle class. This may suggest that working-class women are more prepared to acknowledge publicly that violence has occurred in their marriage. Interestingly, these findings bear close comparison with a similar American study. In 1966, Levinger reported that in a study of divorcing couples 32 per cent of middle-class and 40 per cent of working-class couples mentioned 'physical' abuse as a major complaint (Levinger 1966).

It is estimated that on current trends a third of all marriages currently taking place will end in divorce (Haskey 1982). Assuming that approximately 40 per cent of those will report some violence during their marriage, one can make a rough prediction that two out of five of these marriages will have experienced some physical violence. To these must be added marriages that will not end in divorce, but hold together through periods of possible violence. There may well be as many of these as there are those that will divorce. It is therefore plausible to suggest that something in the region of one in five to one in three of all marriages might experience episodes of physical violence at some point in their history.

Calculations such as these do not, of course, give any indication of the frequency or severity of violence. Although they may represent the more extreme cases, it is salutary to consider the reported experience of women who have escaped to refuges. The Dobash study of 109 women who had used Scottish refuges found that:

'41 per cent of the women experienced their first violent attack within six months after the wedding and another 18 per cent within the first year. Another 25 per cent were hit within the next two years, making a total of 84 per cent within the first three years of marriage. Only 8 per cent of the women did not experience their first attack until after five years of marriage.' (Dobash and Dobash 1979:94)

They also suggest that as the marriage goes on, so the severity of violence may increase, so that by the time the women sought help from the refuge, a majority claimed to have experienced a violent attack by their husbands at least twice a week. A quarter of their sample reported that the violent episode lasted for more than forty-five minutes, the violence being most likely to occur between the hours of 10.00 p.m. and 12.00 a.m. Most of the women reported attacks usually occurring on Friday and Saturday nights, although a significant minority of the sample reported that violence could occur on any day of the week and at any time. The Dobashes further report that most of these violent episodes were preceded by arguments, and, according to the women, the most likely subject of these altercations 'related primarily to the husband's expectations regarding his wife's domestic work, his possessiveness and sexual jealousy and allocation of the family's resources' (1979:95).

Binney, Harkell, and Nixon studied 636 women living in 128 refuges in England and Wales in September 1978. They report that 'not only was the violence these women had suffered severe, but that it had often gone on for a considerable length of time. The average length of time women had suffered was seven years, ranging from a few months to forty years' (1981:5). Forty-seven per cent of their sample had experienced periodic violence for more than six years.

Since there has been no representative study of modern marriage in the United Kingdom, there is no empirical evidence to indicate the prevalence of violence in marriages as a whole. There is, however, an American study that claims to be representative and, on the face of it, has produced some startling findings (Gelles 1979). In 1976 Gelles, Straus, and Steimetz interviewed a representative cross-section of 2,143 American couples. Ten per cent of these couples reported that some form of physical violence had occurred during the previous year of their marriage. They also found that men were more likely to be assaulted than women. Gelles reports that:

> 'When men were asked if they were victims of severe violence, 4.9 per cent said yes. When women were asked if they abused their husbands 4.2 per cent said yes. In terms of violence which could be considered wife abuse 4 per cent of the women said they were abused, while 3.4 per cent of the husbands acknowledged committing severe acts of violence.' (Gelles 1979:140)

Whatever the validity of these American findings, they should perhaps make us cautious about assuming that women are far more likely than men to be victims of marital violence. The fact is that we just do not know whether this is so. But we certainly do know that women are far more likely to seek help because of violence. There are studies of homicide and criminal assault that point overwhelmingly to the preponderance of female victims (Gibson and Klein 1969; McClintock 1963).

It should also be remembered that most British evidence of marital violence comes from agency reports. It would be wrong to assume that the people who seek help from these agencies are the ones most likely to be involved in marital violence. They are merely the cases that practitioners know about. Letitia Allen has shown how in the case of child abuse, knowledge of welfare cases skews estimates of prevalence. She points to the dangers of assuming that the poor who most often use these services are the ones most likely to abuse children (Allen 1978). Similarly, women in financial hardship who are victims of marital violence may be more driven to seek the help of statutory and voluntary welfare agencies and refuges. In this respect it is worth noting that Binney, Harkell, and Nixon (1981) showed that women using refuges came predominantly from local authority housing.

Notes

1 The available information about these 105 cases (less identifying names and addresses) was transferred on to a specially designed card. This recorded information on: the sex of the client, their marital state, whether there were children, whether violence was the main reason for the client approaching the Bureau, the date when the client came to the Bureau, who the original informant was, the nature of the violence complained of, and what action the Bureau took.
2 In our feasibility study we also approached staff at Frenchay Hospital, to the north-east of the city. We were told that as their accident department dealt almost exclusively with road casualties, it would not be worthwhile collecting information about cases of marital violence. We therefore excluded this hospital from our investigation.
3 Collection was discontinued at the Bristol Royal Infirmary after the sister-in-charge changed her job.
4 These calculations are based on 'new' cases, excluding patients returning for further treatment.
5 Four part-time health visitors were excluded from these calculations.
6 See Farragher (1981). By observing policemen attending domestic incidents, Farragher has studied at first hand the way police constables exercise their discretion. He shows the factors at work which contribute to the relatively low prosecution rate.
7 A three-year research project (1979-81) conducted in the Department of Social Administration, University of Bristol, and funded by the Joseph Rowntree Memorial Trust. We are grateful to our colleagues Gwynn Davis and Alison Macleod for giving their permission for us to quote these data.

3
Some social characteristics of victims of marital violence

Despite the possibility that as many as one in three marriages may experience episodes of violence, there is a paucity of information about their social characteristics. This is partly because marital violence is a largely hidden phenomenon and the marriages concerned are consequently not easily identifiable. But even when they do come to the notice of public services, little information is collected about them; and curiously, some of the recent studies of women who use refuges have produced little information of this kind (Dobash and Dobash 1979; Binney, Harkell, and Nixon 1981).

In an attempt to make up for this deficiency we asked the four practitioner groups in our main survey, plus the hospital accident departments, Bristol Marriage Guidance, and the Catholic Marriage Advisory Council – who took part in our Agency Study – to record some basic information about victims who sought their help.[1] Agency case records are usually confined to details about how the case is dealt with, how it is referred, what the presenting problems or injuries are, what help, advice, or treatment is offered, and how long contact with the service is maintained. Very little social information is routinely recorded. We found that the only standard item collected was age. However, in the case studies obtained from our practitioner sample, we were able to record useful additional information about length of marriage, family size, socio-economic status, and agency use and referral. We thus divided our collection of case studies into two groups according to the amount of social information available. The first, and most useful, comprised 128 completed by solicitors, social workers, health visitors, and general medical practitioners. The second group of seventy-one cases was obtained from the intake monitoring survey carried out by the hospital accident departments and the marriage guidance councils.

The individual totals of cases received from each sample were as follows:

Case Sample One
(n = 128)

Solicitors 29
Local authority social workers 34
Health visitors 40
GPs 25

Case Sample Two
(n = 71)

Hospital accident depts 55
Marriage Guidance Councils 16

Sex of victim

In 94 per cent of Case Sample One the victim was female. In the remaining 6 per cent of cases, both partners were mentioned as being victims of the other. In Case Sample Two there was only one male victim, the remainder being women, except for five cases where both partners were injured.

Age of victim

Figure 3(1) plots the age distribution of the victims using a quinquennial (five-year interval) scale for those under forty and a decimal (ten-year interval) scale for the remainder. As a basis for comparison the age distribution of divorcing women is also plotted using data published in the 1976 Marriage and Divorce Statistics (OPCS 1979).

Both samples are fairly closely correlated. Women in their late twenties and early thirties predominate, a finding in line with Pahl's (1978) study of women attending the Canterbury refuge and NWAF's larger study (1981) of 636 women drawn from 128 refuges in England and Wales. In Case Sample One, 80 per cent of the women known to health visitors and 67 per cent of those known to social workers were under the age of thirty-six. The respective figure for women under thirty-six known to solicitors and GPs was 48 per cent. The corresponding data concerning male partners of the victims are 65 per cent and 52 per cent respectively for the health visitor and social worker samples and 37 per cent and 32 per cent for the solicitors and GPs. Fifty-seven per cent of the women going to hospital accident departments were under thirty-six, as were 50 per cent of those going to Marriage Guidance, although our samples here are too small to be reliable.

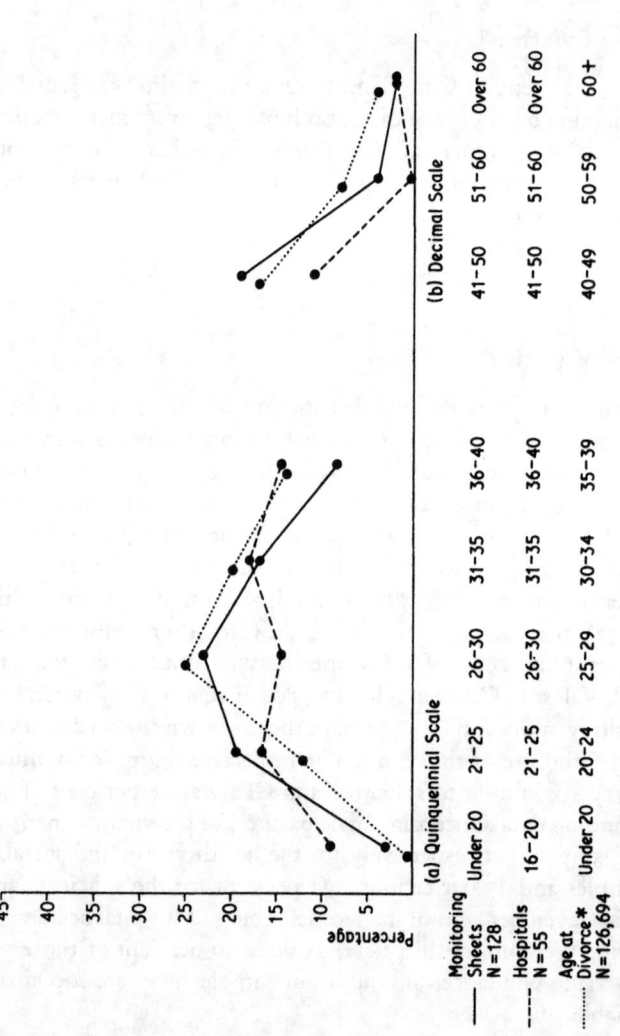

Figure 3(1) *Age of victims of marital violence (case monitoring study and hospital patients) compared with divorcing women*

Length of marriage or cohabitation

In Case Sample One, sixteen of the 128 women were reported as cohabiting. One was divorced and living on her own. In six cases the marital status was not given, and the remaining 105 were listed as married. Of these, eleven (or 8 per cent of the sample) were in their second marriage.

Practitioners were asked to state the length of the marriage or cohabitation if this was known. *Table 3(1)* gives the results of this question.

Table 3(1) *Length of current marriage or cohabitation. Case Sample One (n = 128)*

Years	%
0– 4	22
5– 9	29
10–14	18
15–19	11
20–24	8.5
25–29	2
30+	4
Not known	5.5

Most cases arose within the first ten years of marriage. Most of the cases reported by health visitors (70 per cent) and social workers (63 per cent) came within this group. By contrast the majority, 72 per cent of doctors' cases and 55 per cent of the lawyers' cases, had been living together for more than ten years. This is the kind of distribution one would expect, bearing in mind the statutory duties that health visitors and social workers have for young families. Even so, it is a little puzzling that doctors should report so many longer term partnerships.[2] Further sampling would be needed to evaluate the significance of this finding.

Children of the 'marital' partnership

All practitioners were asked to indicate how many children their patient/client had, and to give details of the children's ages. *Table 3(2)* gives details about family size.

Of these families there were forty (31 per cent) with one child under five, twenty-one (16 per cent) with two children under five, and four

Table 3(2) *Family composition, Case Sample One (n = 128)*

	Total all groups %	Solicitor (n = 29) %	Social worker (n = 34) %	Health visitor (n = 40) %	GP (n = 25) %
Childless	3.1	7	–	–	8
1 child family	18.0	21	15	23	12
2	34.0	28	35	33	44
3	24.2	24	18	27	28
4	10.2	10	18	10	–
5+	10.2	10	15	7	8

(3 per cent) with three under-fives. In other words, in the total sample 50 per cent of the couples had children under five years old. This masks the preponderance of cases reported by social workers and health visitors who work predominantly with young families. Thus, 77 per cent of the couples known to the health visitors and 53 per cent of those known to the social workers had children under five compared with respective figures of 41 per cent for the solicitors and 32 per cent for the doctors.

Socio-economic status

It proved too difficult to gather uniform data about the socio-economic status of the services' clientele. Most of the women were not in paid employment, usually because they were looking after small children. In about one-third of Case Sample One practitioners were unable to give us any information about the husbands' occupations. The data that we obtained were therefore too imprecise to be of much use. Nevertheless, our impression was that there was a fairly general spread broadly comparable to the distribution of the socio-economic spectrum. The data shows some weighting in favour of the lower socio-economic categories, but this may merely reflect a bias in the clientele of the referring agencies, particularly the Social Services Department, and families known to the health visitors where parents will be young. Further evidence to support the relationship between socio-economic status and agency use is given by Binney, Harkell, and Nixon (1981), who show that 75 per cent of the women in refuges came from local authority housing. Rightly, they point out that this does not necessarily mean that marital violence is more common amongst local authority tenants, but rather that women from owner-occupied homes, who may be wealthier, may have access to a wider range of housing solutions.

Since it is known that the divorcing population does not differ markedly in terms of the husband's occupation from that of the still married population (Murch 1980; Gibson 1974), it is possible to compare the data we have gathered with other published information of the divorcing population, as shown in *Table 3(3)*.

Table 3(3) *Socio-economic distribution of husband's occupation*

	n = 88 (adjusted to exclude 40 cases where relevant data were not available) %		1966 Divorcing* %	
Professional (I)	2	} 9	}	12
Intermediate (II)	6			
Skilled Non-manual (III NM)	7	} 46	}	55
Skilled Manual (III M)	33			
Partly Skilled (IV)	10	} 45	}	33
Unskilled (V)	30			

* Registrar General's 1967 Statistical Review.

Agency use and referral

Finally in this chapter we report some data that we have gathered from our case studies concerning the use clients make of services. When giving details of the most recent case of marital violence they had dealt with, practitioners were asked to state whether they knew if the client/patient had already sought help about the marital problem from any other service. *Table 3(4)* classifies their replies.

This table should be interpreted with caution. It is not a reliable indicator of the pattern of agency use in such cases. Practitioners are generally only involved at one moment of a couple's matrimonial history. Some, such as doctors, are more likely to be involved in the earlier stages of breakdown while others, such as lawyers, may be

Table 3(4) *Whether client known to have sought help from other services*

Services contacted	Solicitors (n = 29) %	Social workers (n = 34) %	Health visitors (n = 40) %	GPs (n = 25) %
Solicitor	(–)	32	20	36
Social worker	17	(–)	30	32
Health visitor	3	35	(–)	24
General practitioner	41	47	47	(–)
Marriage Guidance	14	9	7	4
Police	51	29	25	32
Clergy	7	3	2	–

Note: The percentages in these columns refer to the proportion in each sample mentioning contact with a particular service.

brought in nearer the end. In general we agree with the Dobashes' (1979) hypothesis that

> 'As the violent episodes increase in frequency and severity injuries become worse, silence becomes more difficult and dangerous to maintain and different types of help are needed, the intimate and informal sources of assistance are augmented by the more formal social agencies.'

Nevertheless, in our study we have insufficient information to chart the typical patterns of agency use during the history of marriage breakdown. But even relying on reports from practitioners, it is noticeable how frequently certain services were mentioned. General practitioners top the list, followed by the police, solicitors, and social workers. (It is likely that some solicitors forgot to mention that their client was in touch with a health visitor.) These appear to be key services for this population. On this evidence, Marriage Guidance was referred to markedly less often than the other main services. We shall consider the question of the significance of agency choice more fully in Chapter 12.

Referral

Practitioners were also asked: 'Did you refer the client to any other service or agency? If yes, to which?'. *Table 3(5)* classifies the replies.

Social characteristics of victims 37

Table 3(5) *Individual case studies referral pattern (percentaged for comparison)*

Agencies referred to	Solicitors (n = 29) %	Social workers (n = 34) %	Health visitors (n = 40) %	GPs (n = 25) %
Solicitor	(–)	20	25	12
Social worker	7	(–)	35	–
Health visitor	–	–	(–)	8
General practitioner	–	3	22	(–)
Marriage Guidance	7	3	15	8
Police	3	–	–	4
Clergy	–	–	2	–

It was striking that health visitors referred more than any other practitioners, mostly using social workers, solicitors, and general practitioners. Solicitors referred least but were the main referral point for social workers and general practitioners. Relatively few cases were referred to Marriage Guidance, most coming from health visitors. It is remarkable that not one made any reference to Bristol Women's Aid or to women's refuges in general, bearing in mind that they were all cases of marital violence.

Notes

1 We did not do this in the case of some of the smaller agencies, such as the Avon Council on Alcoholism, because the intake survey suggested that they dealt with insufficient numbers. The Citizens Advice Bureau did not take note of the age, occupation, or length of marriage of their clientele, and it was not possible for them to undertake a special survey for us. We did not seek this information from the police since more detailed studies of their involvement with domestic violence were being undertaken at the Universities of Keele and Stirling.
2 In Chapter 12, which considers the significance of agency choice, we offer some possible explanation for this. Since doctors are primarily turned to by people who are committed to the continuance of marriage, this finding may reflect the possibility that there are many middle-aged and older women who have experienced violence but have decided to put up with it and not seek separation or divorce. In our opinion, of all public services, doctors are the most likely to encounter this group of women.

PART II

In this Part we focus on practitioners' individual perceptions of, and response to, marital violence. In this context we consider how they define it, explain it, and acquire evidence to substantiate it. We examine the problem of privacy which makes the practitioners' acquisition of reliable information difficult and which may contribute to ambivalence in practitioners and victims. We then consider two aspects of the practitioners' knowledge base that determine their response: first, their understanding of the law, and second, their understanding of the extent and limits of their own role and those of practitioners in other services.

4
Problems of definition

'I wouldn't call it physical violence. He hit me once or twice. He used to give me a bash. Nothing serious. Just temper. He used to just give me a good whack across the face or something like that. Oh, yes – I didn't like it but – it's a thing of the past now. I wouldn't have it from anybody else, let's put it that way, but I was married. It wasn't continuous, it wasn't every day or anything.'
(Housewife. Age: 41. Divorced and living with new partner. Two children in the care of former husband. Length of marriage: 19 years)

Introduction

Interviewer: 'How would you define marital violence?'
Doctor: 'Any aggressive, hostile behaviour which falls outside the normal rough and tumble of marriage.'

Marital violence is an extraordinarily imprecise term (Miller 1975; Gelles 1973). A general practitioner would probably not say to a health visitor: 'You had better visit Mrs Smith because she is a victim of marital violence'. He would be more likely to say, 'because her husband has blacked her eye, threatened her, or she says he pushed her down the stairs'. These are precise descriptions of behaviour. By contrast the term 'marital violence' embraces a wide range of behaviour. It was our task to discover what behaviour practitioners considered was encompassed by a term that policy makers, government departments, and researchers are increasingly using.

Method of approach

In approaching the problem of definition, we used a series of vignettes covering a range of behaviour that might be regarded as violent. Practitioners were asked which they would include within their own definition. This approach adapted one used by Gelles (1973) and

Straus (1977), who classified behaviour on a scale of increasing severity. The disadvantage of a scale is that it is almost impossible to avoid introducing some subjective element in the weighting. We therefore converted the mechanism of scale into a sieve. This distinguished behaviour that practitioners included in their definition from behaviour that they did not include. The vignettes were matched in five pairs to allow for both husband-wife and wife-husband violence. The resulting order was then rearranged so that it did not suggest an obvious progressive scale of severity. (It might have been wiser to separate the pairs and avoid any implication that they should be treated alike.)

The list was as follows:

1 Angry husband punches wife and breaks her nose.
2 Angry wife wounds husband with broken bottle.
3 Husband shoves wife who has insulted him.
4 Wife slaps husband who has insulted her.
5 Husband frightens wife by threatening to wound her.
6 Wife threatens husband with knife.
7 Husband taunts wife about poor housekeeping.
8 Wife refuses to talk to husband for six months.
9 Husband makes sexual demands of wife which he knows she finds repugnant, and forces her to comply.
10 Wife, angry because husband drinks too much, hits him with poker when he returns from pub.

Having made their selection, practitioners were asked to give a definition of marital violence. Their verbatim replies were recorded.

The form of definition

Practitioners used three kinds of definition. The most common were those based on the form of the behaviour itself, usually determined by whether or not it involved physical force or threats. Second were those based on the consequences suffered by the victim, for example whether or not an actual injury had been sustained or whether the victim had been frightened. Third, some practitioners formulated their definition according to the kinds of response they felt they could offer their client. For example, one lawyer said: 'My professional definition is governed by the remedies available. My test then is, what is needed for an injunction or a divorce?' We should also point out that most practitioners used the term 'marital violence' pejoratively. Only a few used it simply descriptively. Social values therefore played an important part in the way definitions were formulated (see Campbell 1976). Furthermore, it was clear that some practitioners used standards that they would apply to their own lives, while others used those that they perceived as relevant to those of their clients. For example, one doctor said: 'It's not so much what I think – it's what the patients define as violence. I must beware of judging what's normal for them by what's normal for me'. A solicitor remarked: 'I wouldn't have an absolute criterion. It depends on the client's definition – on what they are prepared to put up with'.

The criteria used

The criteria that practitioners used when working out a definition of marital violence need to be distinguished.

USE OF FORCE

Some practitioners restricted violence to physical force; others did not, e.g:

'I would include any situation where either party uses physical force. I would ignore whether it's justified. I would not include verbal abuse, although that forms part of most unreasonable behaviour divorce petitions.' (Solicitor)

'I see it as any violent act leading to injury as opposed to a mere threat.' (Social Worker)

Others included nagging, shouting, and other kinds of verbal intimidation. Some of these based their definition on whether or not the victim became fearful or demoralized. For example, one solicitor remarked: 'One of the worst forms of violence is persistent intellectual bullying by the more intelligent partner'.

INJURY

One doctor said: 'My definition is whether there is actual injury'. Similarly, a health visitor remarked: 'I would only call it marital violence if it involved real injury'.

SEVERITY

> 'Violence has to be serious, involving risk of injury. Shoves and slaps are normal and not serious. The degree of severity is the test.' (Doctor)

> 'I'm only concerned with serious injury. There's a little violence in many marriages, that's only to be expected. A lot of people are quick tempered and slap and shove, but that's not real marital violence.' (Health Visitor)

While it is quite clear that this practitioner had some kind of severity test in mind, her actual use of words is curious. She uses violence in a precise way (slapping, shoving) and the term 'marital' is added to mean 'severe'.

FREQUENCY

A health visitor remarked: 'I wouldn't include many situations if they occurred only once. But if it's repeated until it becomes a set pattern of behaviour then it becomes marital violence'. A solicitor explained that in his view 'real marital violence' was persistent[1] physical abuse:

> 'The worst cases are those women who are worn out by violence, not necessarily extreme severe violence, but the almost continual pushing, shoving, and threatening which makes you keep your mouth shut. It undermines them. It's persistence that drives them to distraction, they're so demoralized. They become doormats.'

INTENT

For some, intent was important. For example, a social worker thought that there had to be a clear intention 'to do serious harm'. Also those using the legitimacy criterion (see below) were by implication taking account of the 'assailant's' intention. But the majority of practitioners seemed to exclude intention from their definition. This may be an intuitive recognition that pent emotion which finds expression in violence often contains a large unconscious element.

NORMALITY

The key variable in terms of whether or not given behaviour is included in the practitioner's definition is the word 'marital', not 'violence'. The test thus becomes: what is acceptable behaviour within marriage? The emphasis is placed on the word 'marital' rather than on the word 'violence'. Practitioners who sought to exclude 'normal behaviour' from their definition of marital violence were nearly always using it in a pejorative sense. For example, a social worker told us: 'It has to be intended use of physical force or threat of it. Slaps are used quite often but I would exclude slapping on the basis that it's normal'. One health visitor remarked: 'Wordy battles and arguments are not real violence. That's normal in marriage'.

TOLERATION

Another test sometimes applied was whether the victim could tolerate violence. One health visitor remarked:

'All these situations would fall within my own personal definition. I don't believe anyone has the right to act in any of these ways to anyone. Yet some people would accept it – they like a bit of drama in their marriage. It all depends on their level of tolerance and on their expectations.'

A solicitor commented: 'There are some couples where one might say the relationship is enriched by physical violence, but that is consensual'. This practitioner was referring to the toleration level of a couple rather than an individual, suggesting that each relationship has its own standard.

LEGITIMACY

Some practitioners excluded from their definitions behaviour they considered to be justified or legitimate. For example, one practitioner remarked that in his view there were circumstances, such as a discovered infidelity, 'where violence is right, and where I would be surprised if the aggrieved partner was not violent' (Doctor). Many practitioners used the expression 'unprovoked violence' as if provocation divested the behaviour of its pejorative character, for example:

'It has to be unprovoked aggression, a direct physical assault, leading to physical injury. It seems there's often good reason for the violence – the woman tries her husband's patience. Sometimes they do it to cause excitement in their dull lives. Some women enjoy it and almost seem to need it.' (Health Visitor)

SOCIAL CONTEXT

A few practitioners thought that the social context within which the behaviour occurred could be the key element in determining its inclusion in their definition. This test was nearly always used in combination with the toleration test, but it should be distinguished in its own right because it is so obviously different. Behaviour labelled 'marital violence' in one social context was not so in another. In each instance, the practitioner assumed that middle-class families would be less tolerant of aggressive behaviour than working-class ones. Here are several examples:

> 'Under certain circumstances violence which personally seems to me to be wrong under *any* circumstances is accepted in some of the marriages on the X (well-known council estate) where I work.' (Doctor)

> 'What would be acceptable to a family in Y (another working-class district) wouldn't be acceptable in middle-class marriages.' (Solicitor)

> 'I come from a Jewish background where this kind of behaviour would be incredible. I was very shocked initially when I started to practise, but I've come to accept it as normal in many families now.' (Doctor)

COMBINATION TESTS

Many practitioners used some kind of combination test, taking into account several factors such as the degree of severity, frequency, and even the effect on the victim. It may be that cases judged to be less serious require a combination of factors to justify inclusion in the practitioner's definition. Here are four examples, each with a different combination:

1 *Physical force, intent, and normality*

> 'Physical assault with intent to do physical damage or where they threaten in a way which I would consider is no normal threat. It has to arouse fear.' (Social Worker)

2 *Frequency and severity*

> 'Either repeated minor violence like slapping, pinching, or punching provided it's not too powerful, or a single episode of serious violence using weapons or heavy punching.' (Doctor)

3 Frequency, intent, and effect on victim

'It has to be continuous – a sudden outburst can happen in any marriage. The intention is important. Prolonged mental cruelty is as injurious as physical attack.' (Health Visitor)

4 Frequency and effect on victim

'There must be a continuing situation in a cruel worked-up state, not just an isolated blow or shove. The other person also has to be frightened of it.' (Social Worker)

Variations between occupations

At first sight it seems alarming that there are so many different views about what constitutes marital violence. People may fail to appreciate how varied each other's definitions are. In order to see how serious a problem this could be, we quantified the answers to our vignettes in order to gauge the extent of the variation (*Tables 4(1)* and *4(2)* below). It will be seen that while there was general agreement that wounding should be included, there was serious disagreement about

Table 4(1) *High inclusion rate (70% +) × occupation*

Situation	Total all occupations (n = 200) %	Solicitors (n = 50) %	Social workers (n = 50) %	Health visitors (n = 50) %	GPs (n = 50) %
Husband punches wife – breaks nose	97	100	98	92	96
Wife wounds husband with bottle	97	98	98	94	96
Wife hits husband with poker	89	96	88	80	90
Husband forces wife to have sex	82	86	90	78	72
Husband threatens to wound wife	82	92	78	78	80
Wife threatens husband with knife	81	86	78	78	82

48 Marital Violence

Table 4(2) *Moderate to low inclusion rate (46% and below)* × *occupation*

Situation	Total all occupations (n = 200) %	Solicitors (n = 50) %	Social workers (n = 50) %	Health visitors (n = 50) %	GPs (n = 50) %
Wife slaps husband	38	46	28	44	38
Husband shoves wife	37	46	24	36	38
Wife refuses to talk to husband	31	18	34	36	34
Husband taunts wife	22	12	22	30	22

Table 4(3) *Husband shoves wife – whether included or excluded* × *occupation*

	Total all occupations (n = 200) %	Solicitors (n = 50) %	Social workers (n = 50) %	Health visitors (n = 50) %	GPs (n = 50) %
Include + if repeated	37	46	28	36	38
Exclude	48	38	60	46	48
Do not know	14	16	12	18	10
No response	1	–	–	–	4

Table 4(4) *Wife slaps husband – whether included or excluded* × *occupation*

	Total all occupations (n = 200) %	Solicitors (n = 50) %	Social workers (n = 50) %	Health visitors (n = 50) %	GPs (n = 50) %
Include + if repeated	38	46	24	44	38
Exclude	47	38	62	40	46
Do not know	14	16	14	16	12
No response	1	–	–	–	4

slaps and shoves (*Tables 4(3)* and *4(4)*), and a tendency to exclude those situations that did not involve physical force or threats (*Tables 4(5)* and *4(6)*).

Table 4(5) *Husband taunts wife – whether included or excluded × occupation*

	Total all occupations (n = 200) %	Solicitors (n = 50) %	Social workers (n = 50) %	Health visitors (n = 50) %	GPs (n = 50) %
Include + if repeated	22	12	22	30	22
Exclude	68	86	72	54	60
Do not know	8	2	6	16	12
No response	2	–	–	–	6

Table 4(6) *Wife refuses to talk to husband for six months – whether included or excluded × occupation*

	Total all occupations (n = 200) %	Solicitors (n = 50) %	Social workers (n = 50) %	Health visitors (n = 50) %	GPs (n = 50) %
Include + if repeated	31	18	34	36	34
Exclude	57	76	60	40	52
Do not know	10	6	4	22	10
No response + other	2	–	2	2	4

It is remarkable that there was no consensus about even the most common category, that of the husband who punched his wife and broke her nose.

There are discernible differences between occupational groups. For example, a comparatively high number of solicitors (twenty-three) included slapping and shoving compared with social workers (fourteen and twelve) (*Tables 4(3)* and *4(4)*). Health visitors were more likely than solicitors to include taunting husbands and silent wives (*Tables 4(5)* and *4(6)*). It is hard to explain such differences. It may be that solicitors are guided by the kinds of behaviour that courts will accept as proof for divorce petitions or injunctions. Health visitors and GPs have the closest similarity. It could well be that when everyone is so woolly about definitions, practitioners' ability to take action will colour their definition.

Discussion

Our evidence suggests the following propositions: first, that practitioners differ in what kinds of behaviour they define as 'marital violence'; second, the less severe the physical consequences for the victim the less likely it is that the behaviour will be included in the practitioner's definition; third, that the term 'marital violence' is more often than not used pejoratively,[2] and if behaviour is regarded as normal it is much less likely to be condemned. Also, the term 'marital violence', in so far as it is used at all by practitioners, acts as a blanket expression covering a wide range of behaviour. It is imprecise and ambiguous, with the consequence that people can easily think they are talking about the same thing when in fact they are not.

We think marital violence is an inadequate term. If anyone should be called to account for using it, it is the policy makers and researchers, who are propagating it by inviting the professional population at large to incorporate it in their vocabulary. Our impression is that practitioners do not like using it in their day-to-day work, probably because it is not particularly functional. You cannot 'marital violence someone'.[3] Since practitioners are always having to describe behaviour in terms of what happened, when and how, the lack of a verb is a real handicap to its use. That may be fortuitous in view of the term's other shortcomings.

The question remains why its use may be spreading. It could be that its very ambiguity serves social and political purposes. Ambiguity and imprecision might conceal the extent of disagreement about whether or not certain kinds of behaviour (for example slapping and shoving) should be socially acceptable. Since the term 'marital violence' seems to be widely regarded as pejorative, people who use it are likely to feel that they share a sense of moral indignation. This may be just what reformers need to arouse if they are to mobilize services for battered women and create new social policies. Shared moral indignation may unite people in a common purpose.

This line of thought has a further consequence. The more a type of behaviour is included within a pejorative blanket term, the more it may lose its social acceptability. This is likely to be the case regardless of whether or not the behaviour is normal and its practice widespread.

This is the way behaviour becomes socially proscribed. It is as if the blanket term contaminates one type of behaviour, previously regarded as acceptable, by linking it with another that is not. Once behaviour is proscribed in this way its practice may eventually become less widespread and hence less normal. Thus the effect of the pejorative character of the blanket is to widen the range of socially unacceptable behaviour. This illustrates how particular forms of behaviour may be defined variously and modified at different times in our social history as the currency of social values alters.

In considering questions of definition we have come to realize how words structure people's thoughts and perceptions.[4] Developing technical language may condition thoughts and responses. It may have profound effects on people's behaviour. This is no mere academic point. For example, in the expression '*victim* of marital violence', the word 'victim' may arouse a response in rather the same way as dogs salivated when they heard Pavlov's bell. Researchers may salivate similarly, and may accordingly be more open to criticism than most.

Notes

1 We observe that practitioners who used this test practically always assumed that the violence was unilateral, perpetrated by the man on the woman. Of course, there may well be partnerships where there are frequent rows in which each 'fights' the other, but these were seldom if ever mentioned in this context.
2 The expression 'marital violence' may be used as a simple description of behaviour. More often than not, however, one could deduce from the context in which the phrase was used that the respondent was implying social or moral disapproval as well, hence our use of the adverb 'pejoratively'.
3 It is worth noting that the same point applies to the word 'violence'. You have to *do* violence to something or someone. The verb 'to violate' has a variety of meanings. The Penguin English Dictionary suggests: 'to rape'; 'to brutally destroy or disturb'; 'to treat (something holy) with disrespect'. This last definition is interesting in the context of marital violence, since it could be used to imply that in marriage and other close domestic relationships disrespect shown by one partner to the other is a violation of the person or the institution of marriage. Some of our respondents who used a broad definition of the term marital violence may have meant something of this kind.
4 In making this point we should, perhaps, acknowledge the converse argument that perceptions influence word choice, but this is not relevant to the argument that we develop here.

5
Problems of explanation

'She tried to kill me, smashed a bottle at me, went for me with a knife, threw an alarm clock. Mind, I asked for it, I got her to such a pitch of annoyance. And I had to hit her. She wouldn't stop nagging and I could have killed her, but I'm not proud of it – I was ashamed of carrying on like that.'
(Lorry Driver. Age: 34. Divorced. 2 children in care of mother. Length of marriage: 15 years)

'He hit me quite often but it was more mental than physical. He always used to suffer from these moods, but you couldn't say how often they happened. He was the type of man who let things get him down. We didn't have a very good sex life and he let this play on his mind and he'd go to bed for months, literally months, and only get up to make himself a cup of tea, nothing else.'
(Housewife. Age: 45. Divorced. 1 child in her care. Length of marriage: 25 years)

Introduction

Most studies of marital violence conclude that its causes are not really understood (e.g. Gelles 1972; Steimetz and Straus 1974). In any particular case a whole range of theories may be used to explain violence. These have been well summarized by Freeman (1979: 127-50), and the Dobashes (1979). Although the Parliamentary Select Committee urged that there should be research into causes, we felt that that would be too ambitious an undertaking. In so far as we were investigating the phenomenon of violence between partners we were doing so through an intervening and distorting lens. We set out to examine how this lens works. In this Chapter, our concern is with the practitioner's view of violence between partners, and explanations for it. Sometimes, as we shall see, such views suggest that there may be a correlation between marital violence and certain facts in the couple's social or psychological background. We know of no scientific studies that have been able to validate correlations of this kind.[1] In effect, we have been studying what practitioners believe, rather than know, to be the causes of marital violence.

It is difficult to know how best to present our findings because a great many issues come within its scope. They do not readily fall into a pattern or line of argument. Three general questions are raised by our material: first, whether practitioners feel they need to explain marital violence to themselves when they encounter it; second, what sorts of explanations they favour most; third, what purposes both the choice and form of their explanations serve. In our attempts to create a coherent, overall picture, we use threads of general ideas and theories to fix onto a backcloth the bits and pieces of material that illustrate individual practitioners' explanations.

Marsden has pinpointed an important difficulty concerning the use of explanations. He calls it the problem of the 'vocabulary of motives', by which he means that people caught up in violent partnerships, and outsiders who have dealings with them, often have different motives from each other when explaining violence to themselves and other audiences. His point is that people tailor their explanations to suit the response they are seeking from others. He writes that:

> 'explanations may be volunteered or omitted as individuals sense their acceptability. Moreover it seems that people with a particular definition of their own problem will tend to approach those agencies which most nearly fit the definition. For example if a problem is seen as psychiatric, a psychiatrist may be approached, or if seen as sheer bullying, the police. There may thus develop a self confirming, self selection of particular kinds of cases, offering particular kinds of emotional accounts, approaching the selected agencies which are most likely to accept and confirm those accounts.' (Marsden 1978)

We had to bear this consideration in mind when we asked practitioners for their explanations. We also recognized that people may well seek explanations that confirm their own image of themselves. Despite this, it would be unwise to assume that practitioners' perceptions of violence between partners have no value because inevitably they are distorted and selective.

By bringing together the observations of practitioners we may find clues that will eventually help policy makers and practitioners better understand why people behave violently towards their partners. By identifying factors believed to be associated with violent behaviour, it may be possible to isolate the elements that have a causal connection. This might lead to better understanding of what could be done both to prevent its occurrence and to help those whose lives are damaged by it. At the moment we are a long way from this. The material reported in this chapter is more relevant to our understanding of the responses and views of the practitioners themselves.

Method of approach

We studied practitioners' explanations in two ways. First they were invited to generalize by being asked:

> 'Do you have any views about factors which may precipitate marital violence? By precipitate we do not necessarily mean cause.'

Second, they were invited to particularize by being asked what factors they thought might have precipitated the violence in the latest case with which they had dealt. (We outline the method by which these case studies were obtained in the Appendix.)

There are weaknesses in this approach. First, it begs all the questions associated with definition discussed in Chapter 4. Second, we acknowledge that by asking practitioners such questions we may have been inviting them to devise explanations for our benefit, when previously they might have had no conscious views at all. Also in the first general question, by emphasizing the word 'precipitate', we may have been encouraging practitioners to concentrate their thoughts on the immediate precipitating factor rather than on their view of the 'real' or 'underlying' reasons. In addition, our interview might have prompted them to think about possible explanations which they later applied to the case selected for us. This is, of course, part of a more general problem inherent in our research, namely that we might well have been raising practitioners' consciousness of marital violence.

Nevertheless, despite these weaknesses, we think our two questions complement each other usefully. The interview question elicited practitioners' general ideas, preconceptions, and stereotyped images of marital violence. The case studies produced material that was more closely related to the reality of their practice. In certain respects, therefore, it was possible to contrast and compare the two sets of information.

The chapter is divided into four parts: the first explains our method of classification; the second presents quantitative data from interviews and case studies; the third contains illustrations from case studies. In the fourth we interpret our findings and discuss some of the questions raised.

Findings

We aimed to classify those explanations that seemed most commonly used. In so doing, we are open to the criticism that our classification is to some extent arbitrary, and may involve some over-simplification.

Method of classification

Practitioners offered explanations or views of precipitating factors, both in interviews and in their case studies. We divided their primary explanations into three basic groups: the first contained factors such as poor housing, poverty, unemployment, or illness, which were believed to provoke stress and frustration, manifested in violence; the second contained explanations locating the cause of violence in the personality of one or both of the partners. Since the influence of alcohol and drugs did not easily fit into either of the other two classifications, sometimes being associated with one, the other, or both, we decided to give it a third category. Thirteen basic types of explanation were listed within these three divisions, see *Table 5(1)*.

These classifications not only cover the range of explanations given by practitioners, they also accord with those most frequently encountered in publications on the subject (Miller, Pain, and Webb 1978;

Table 5(1) *Classification of factors*

Group I – Stress factors	Group II – Personality factors	Group III
1 Illness/handicap/ psychiatric disorders	6 Personality of the man	13 Alcohol and drugs
2 Housing	7 Personality of the woman	
3 Poverty	8 The interaction of both	
4 Unemployment	9 Cultural upbringing and role expectation of one or both	
5 Children	10 'Immaturity' of one or both	
	11 Psycho-sexual problems of one or both	
	12 Inarticulateness – intellectual disparity between man and woman	

Marsden 1978). Authorities vary in what they emphasize. Gayford (1978: 24) and Pizzey (1974), for example, stress individual characteristics of the personalities and the importance of alcohol. Gelles (1972) has suggested that the main causes of violence lie in an adaptation of response to structurally induced stress. Goode (1971) and O'Brien (1971) have offered what might be termed a hybrid explanation that bridges the social/structural and the pathological. In their view, men resort to violence when they feel they lack the skills, talents, and resources to fulfil their cultural expectations of superior patriarchal status, a view incidentally that the Dobashes seem recently to have endorsed (Dobash and Dobash 1979), and one that is favoured by feminist writers. Even so, these hybrid explanations, as Leonard and McLeod (1980) point out, do not explain precisely how cultural and sociological factors interact with individual personal behaviour, a difficulty that may incline policy makers, practitioners, and clinical researchers to favour individual rather than cultural explanations. Explanations based on individual personality are easier to grasp, though not necessarily more accurate. We discuss this proposition later in the light of our findings.

Several points need to be made about the thirteen factors. First, although the list is not exhaustive, it was compiled only after a good deal of preliminary field-work, after examining other investigators' classifications and typologies, and after we found that it fitted our evidence.

Second, it should be noticed that we have not made separate categories for what one might term 'moralist' explanations. By this, we mean behaviour considered to be caused by or associated with notions of moral weakness or corrupt character (May 1978). This was not an oversight. We expected to find practitioners who explained behaviour quite explicitly in ethical/moral rather than in social/psychological terms. Occasionally this was so, but more often moral censure appeared veiled behind social science jargon or quasi-medical diagnoses. For example, heavy drinking was often referred to as if it was an indicator of moral weakness. Certain adjectives and expressions were used ambiguously, so that it was hard to tell whether they were intended to be solely descriptive or technical or whether they implied disapproval. This was particularly so of such terms as 'immature', 'deprived', 'unstable'.

Third, we should explain the way we classified explanations under the heading 'Personality factors' in *Table 5(1)*, Group II. We received a wide range of explanations for, and 'labels' describing, behaviour that

Table 5(2) *Aggregation of personality factors*

Factor	Descriptions of behaviour*
6 Personality of man	'quick temper'; 'aggressiveness'; 'psychopathy'; 'selfishness'; 'domineering'; 'bullying'
7 Personality of woman	'nagging'; 'dominating woman'; 'provocative wife'; 'willing victim' or 'masochism'; 'slovenly'; 'bad housekeeper'; 'feckless'; 'unstable'; 'more assertive role of woman'
8 Interaction of both	'incompatibility'; 'sadomasochism'; 'selfishness of both'; 'clash of culture and social background'; 'six of one and half-a-dozen of the other'; 'it takes two to start a row'
9 Cultural upbringing and role expectations of one or both	'deprived childhood'; 'behaviour modelled upon that of parents'; 'cultural role expectations'
10 Immaturity	'emotionally immature'; 'child-like behaviour'; 'too early for marriage'
11 Psycho-sexual problems of one or both	'sexual problems'; 'morbid jealousy'; 'infidelity'

* Expressions used in this column have been taken from evidence obtained in interviews or case studies. Many recur. We do not endorse their use since they do not necessarily have any intrinsic validity.

could be classified under this heading. *Table 5(2)* shows how we aggregated these under four sub-headings.

Quantitative data from interviews and case studies

GENERAL EXPLANATIONS

Having coded all the replies to our questions according to the thirteenfold classification listed in *Tables 5(1)* and *5(2)* we constructed a series of factor-popularity polls. *Table 5(3)* quantifies the explanations given in the interview sample and compares them with those given in the details of the 128 cases they referred to us.

If there is one correlate that comes up over and over again, it is the link between violence and alcohol. We cannot comment on whether or not that link is causal, but in our opinion there is an overwhelming case for thorough investigation of the subject.

It will be noticed that in *Table 5(3)* there is a marked positional

58 Marital Violence

Table 5(3) *Most popular explanation × occupation*

1 Solicitors

Interview sample (n = 50)	%	Case studies (n = 29)	%
1 Alcohol	62	Alcohol	38
2 Money	44	Psycho-sexual problems	31
3 Psycho-sexual problems	32	Interaction	14
4 Upbringing	26	Children	10
5 Personality of woman	26	Personality of man	7
6 Interaction	22	Money	7
7 Children	20	Inarticulateness	3
8 Personality of man	18	Immaturity	–
9 Illness/handicap	14	Upbringing	–
10 Housing	12	Housing	–
11 Inarticulateness	12	Unemployment	–
12 Unemployment	12	Illness/handicap	–
13 Immaturity	8	Personality of woman	–

2 Social Workers

Interview sample (n = 50)	%	Case studies (n = 34)	%
1 Money	62	Personality of man	35
2 Alcohol	40	Alcohol	32
3 Upbringing	38	Personality of woman	32
4 Psycho-sexual problems	36	Interaction	29
5 Housing	34	Money	23
6 Children	30	Unemployment	15
7 Personality of woman	30	Psycho-sexual problems	15
8 Interaction	28	Illness/handicap	15
9 Unemployment	22	Immaturity	12
10 Personality of man	20	Upbringing	12
11 Immaturity	18	Children	9
12 Inarticulateness	12	Housing	6
13 Illness/handicap	8	Inarticulateness	–

Problems of explanation 59

3 Health Visitors

Interview sample (n = 50)	%	Case studies (n = 40)	%
1 Money	68	Personality of woman	38
2 Illness/handicap	54	Interaction	33
3 Alcohol	54	Alcohol	28
4 Immaturity	48	Psycho-sexual problems	28
5 Children	46	Children	23
6 Psycho-sexual problems	46	Upbringing	23
7 Housing	40	Personality of man	23
8 Upbringing	40	Illness	23
9 Interaction	28	Immaturity	20
10 Personality of woman	24	Money	20
11 Unemployment	22	Inarticulateness	8
12 Inarticulateness	20	Housing	5
13 Personality of man	14	Unemployment	3

4 Doctors

Interview sample (n = 50)	%	Case studies (n = 25)	%
1 Alcohol	90	Alcohol	48
2 Psycho-sexual problems	48	Illness/handicap	40
3 Illness/handicap	40	Interaction	20
4 Money	38	Personality of woman	16
5 Upbringing	36	Psycho-sexual problems	16
6 Children	26	Personality of man	12
7 Interaction	24	Unemployment	8
8 Personality of woman	24	Immaturity	8
9 Immaturity	22	Money	8
10 Personality of man	20	Upbringing	8
11 Unemployment	20	Children	4
12 Housing	10	Inarticulateness	–
13 Inarticulateness	4	Housing	–

Note: The percentages refer to the number of practitioners mentioning a particular explanation. They are more significant for the *order* than for the actual frequency.

disparity concerning certain explanations between the two samples. For example, on average 53 per cent of all practitioners mentioned money in the interview sample but only 14.5 per cent did so in the case studies. In each occupational group, money was placed lower in the case studies than in the interview sample. This suggests that professional people assume, contrary to the evidence of their cases, that marital violence is strongly associated with poverty. The question arises why this is so.

It may be that practitioners were unconsciously dissociating marital violence from their own socio-economic status, since they would not normally consider themselves poor. This may be especially so in the case of doctors and solicitors who would normally have more money and a higher standard of living than social workers and health visitors. Similarly, though to a lesser extent, bad housing and heavy drinking appears more in theory (i.e. in the interview sample) than in practice (i.e. in the case studies).

In general, the evidence suggests that social structural explanations predominate in the interview samples, whereas individual personality explanations predominate in the case studies. In our view this distinction hinges on the question of where moral responsibility for behaviour lies, i.e. with elements in society, or with the individual? Thus in this context illness or handicap may be conceived as a state that overtakes the patient and for which he is not therefore to be held morally responsible. We recognize that this begs an enormous number of questions, some of which were examined by Ian Kennedy in his first Reith Lecture (Kennedy 1981). For all that, our evidence is consistent with the argument that people who do not themselves experience marital violence favour explanations that set them apart from those who do,[2] an idea we elaborate later.

Another remarkable finding is that in the interview sample the personality of the woman consistently rates above the personality of the man as an explanation for the violence. Also, in the case studies health visitors and doctors give a higher rating to the personality of the woman than to that of the man. In spite of the fact that women are nearly always the victims of marital violence, it is they who are described as responsible for it, rather than the man who is the perpetrator (Dobash and Dobash 1979). We also find it odd that in their case studies, health visitors (who are all women) point to the personality of the woman as their main explanation. They also give prominence to 'interaction', which also, of course, implicates the woman. These findings may be partly explained by the fact that health visitors have more dealings with women than men. They may, therefore, be more impressed by the personalities of the women whom they meet than by those of the men they see less often. This argument could also apply to the social workers and doctors, yet they do not emphasize the woman's personality quite so much.

We searched through all two hundred interviews and counted how frequently various descriptions were used in relation to the personality of both men and women. These findings are presented in Table 5(4).

Table 5(4) *Interview sample: descriptions of personality (n = 200, all occupations combined)*

Women	n	%
Personality of women not mentioned	148	74.0
'Provocative'	17	8.5
'Willing victim'	14	7.0
'Changing role of women' – more assertive	7	3.5
'Dominating women'	5	2.5
'Depressed'/'housebound'	5	2.5
'Nagging wives'	3	1.5
Other	1	0.5

Men	n	%
Personality of men not mentioned	164	82.0
'Aggressive', 'bullying', 'domineering'	15	7.5
'Quick tempered'	9	4.5
'Selfish'	4	2.0
Other	8	4.0

Other noticeable differences emerge between the occupations. For example, in the two male-dominated occupational samples (solicitors and especially doctors) alcohol comes top of the list, both in the interview sample and case studies.

It is probable that agency setting influences the relative weighting of some of the explanations. For example, as one would expect, doctors and health visitors give a higher rating to psycho-sexual problems and to stress reaction to illness and handicap more often than solicitors and social workers. Association with agency setting emerges in other ways: for example, health visitors and social workers mentioned poor housing more often than doctors and solicitors, possibly because they visit people's houses more and can assess the quality. Stress provoked by children was mentioned most by those occupations which deal directly with child welfare matters.

The agency bias in the weighting given to explanations tells a story all of its own. There is a tendency for practitioners to redefine problems in terms with which they feel most familiar. It suggests that objectivity may be the first victim. Moreover, the patient or client may be reluctant to challenge the redefinition of the problem if overawed by the practitioner's authority.

SPECIFIC MEDICAL EXPLANATIONS

Depression and other psychiatric illness as precipitating factors

Health visitors and general practitioners were asked whether they thought there were specific psychiatric conditions that might aggravate marital tensions and possibly precipitate violence. *Table 5(5)* summarizes their replies.

Table 5(5) *Interview sample: psychiatric illness as an explanation*

	Health visitors (n = 50) %	GPs (n = 50) %
Not mentioned	48	40
Mentioned	52	60

Paranoid schizophrenic and epileptic conditions were the disorders mentioned most frequently. Forty per cent of the health visitors and 34 per cent of the doctors mentioned the victim's depression, which was believed to frustrate the husband and to trigger physical violence. We were told that these husbands did not appreciate the way depression lowered their wives' capacity to be emotionally responsive and to perform everyday tasks. These observations not only pinpoint the problems of depression and illness, but also lend weight to the studies that suggest that some men feel it appropriate to use physical force when their wives are unresponsive to them or do not match up to their expectations of a woman's domestic responsibilities. It is worth noting that practitioners seemed in this context to expect women to be normally responsive to men, but did not mention men's responsiveness to women. None of these practitioners referred to depression in men as a contributory factor.

The possible influence of medically prescribed drugs

Health visitors and doctors were also asked whether they thought the effects of medically prescribed drugs could precipitate violence. *Table 5(6)* quantifies their replies.

Table 5(6) *Interview sample: Might medically prescribed drugs lead to violence?*

	Health visitors (n = 50) %	GPs (n = 50) %
No	44	46
Not in my experience, but could do	16	4
Yes – specifically	38	26
No opinion offered	2	24

Health visitors seemed more inclined than doctors to associate violence with drugs. Doctors were decidedly coy in answering this question – perhaps understandably, since they do the prescribing.

Eleven health visitors said that they thought tranquillizers, by making patients dull and emotionally unresponsive, could contribute to a potentially violent marital relationship. Seven said that certain kinds of contraceptive pill could also have a similar effect. Five mentioned the possibility that some anti-depressant drugs could make a patient excitable and aggressive.

Although doctors were more cautious about expressing an opinion on these matters, there was no doubt that a number were uneasy about the effects of drugs on behaviour, as can be seen from the following comments:

> 'Reaction patterns are different if drugs are involved in marital cases. I've got to be careful how I qualify this. On the whole drugs produce a diminished awareness, and interfere with normal behaviour and responses. I'm afraid drugs can be more subtle in effect than drink.'

'I try to be careful about drugs and how much I give. But it's so easy to get drugs these days. If they are taken in the prescribed manner they shouldn't have any adverse effect on behaviour.'

'I don't think drugs have that much effect, either for good or bad. They don't have the same effect as alcohol in releasing inhibitions. Nearly always it's the women who take tablets. I do give tranquillizers for marital problems. If they get sleepy they should stop taking them and get a lower dosage. It's up to the patient to take the appropriate dose that doesn't dull the senses.'

'It's the original condition that's most likely to be the cause of violence, not the drugs – that's just an excuse.'

This last comment sums up the attitude of most of the doctors to whom we spoke. We have no way of assessing the validity of this view, but it is worth noting that health visitors seem less sanguine. Parrish has written:

'Anti-anxiety drugs are purely symptomatic in their effects and one must ask oneself whether the "damping down" of the patient's symptoms is the most appropriate form of therapy for a disorder precipitated or aggravated by various emotional, physical or environmental stress.' (Parrish 1971)

We are concerned that there are cases where a man's frustration might be increased by his wife's lack of emotional responsiveness, induced by tranquillizing drugs. We think there is need for a more technical investigation of this matter, since a high proportion of women with marital problems are taking such drugs, particularly librium and valium.

Pregnancy and violence

Occasionally, the case studies indicated that the practitioner believed that the violence started when the wife became pregnant, or shortly after the birth of the first child. For example, one health visitor referred to violence being precipitated by

'tension and emotional upheaval resulting from pregnancy and birth of first child. The mother is prone to depression and is particularly anxious. She had a difficult forceps delivery and fears a second pregnancy. . . . She is too engrossed in the baby to the neglect of her husband who feels irritated and rejected.'

Problems of explanation 65

Even so, there were insufficient cases associating pregnancy with the onset of violence to be statistically significant in our sample. This is rather surprising since a number of authorities have linked the onset of violence to the wife's pregnancy (Gelles 1972, 1975; Marsden and Owen 1975). We have spoken to the Sheffield NWAF research team[3] who have told us that in their study of 656 women using refuges, a high proportion claimed that violence began during or soon after the first pregnancy, very often within the first year of marriage.

Illustrations from case studies

Our illustrations show how we approached the task of classifying practitioners' explanations and how practitioners phrased their answers. Each occupation appears to have a distinctive style. For example, doctors gave the briefest explanations and the simplest descriptions, whereas in general, social workers gave the most involved ones. Solicitors tended to keep speculation about explanation to a minimum, preferring to summarize a pattern of deteriorating relationships in the form of a 'story', reminiscent of the way divorce lawyers used to give brief evidence to the court when presenting undefended divorce petitions prior to the introduction of the Special Procedure (see Elston, Fuller, and Murch 1975).

Although the manner in which they wrote their case studies was in part conditioned by the design of our form and the time practitioners were able to spend completing it, we think the replies can be accepted as a general indicator of the way they structured their thoughts. We have chosen four illustrations from each occupational group.[4] Our classifications are given on the left side of the page, and we have italicized and numerated the corresponding sentences or phrases which, in our opinion, contain explanations.

SOLICITORS

Factors   *Case 1*

[1] Inarticulateness   Wife alleges 'blows to head and body'. Husband,
    of husband   my client, says he 'merely pushed her out of the
[2] Money   way'. There had been deteriorating marital
    problems   situation for some time. *Husband, although an*

educated man, said that wife tied him up in knots verbally and went on at him to the point where his reactions became physical because he was losing the verbal battle.[1] He seems quite content to continue a non-speaking 'she leaves any room as soon as I come in' existence. *He had very severe financial troubles at the time.*[2]

Case 2

[1] Psycho-sexual problems
[2] Interaction

This was a case where there were blows, insults, throwing objects, pushing downstairs, tearing clothes, locking wife out of house, demanding sexual intercourse. Unreasonable behaviour throughout the marriage although there have been periods of comparative peace. Unhappy marriage probably due to:
a) *excessive demands for sexual intercourse* by male respondent;[1]
b) *Respondent preferred to stay at home whereas female Petitioner (client) liked a busy social life;*[2]
c) *jealousy by Respondent.*[1] All leading to abuse, violence, and deterioration of marriage.
d) husband often full of remorse and begs forgiveness in tears.
e) wife left on previous occasions but persuaded against better judgement to return and try to provide a home for children.

Case 3

[1] Alcohol – man
[2] Housing

Occasional physical attacks on wife (client) and on elder boys, but constant name-calling, insulting, *urinating and vomiting in the house following drunken return thereto,*[1] embarrassment to children and their friends. *The wife tolerated violence for many years from 1972 onwards while children were small and she could not get alternative accommodation with such a brood.*[2] She was a Roman Catholic and had a long time squaring her conscience and going for a divorce. We first saw her in 1972. She moved to

Problems of explanation 67

divorce in February 1977. She endured violence for longer than was necessary because she had been told by local housing authority she could not be provided with alternative accommodation because her family was too numerous and all were adequately housed. We advised application to the Magistrate's Court, and obtained Legal Aid to enable her to do so, to obtain custody of children to add weight to her application for housing, but she would not allow us to issue summons when all was prepared.

Case 4

[1] Interaction – possibly personality of both

Client (wife) struck and pushed about. Precipitating incident was husband setting fire to some furniture. This was an isolated incident to the extent that nothing like it had happened before. This lady was, at least in my office and at court, particularly self-controlled and objective about her problems. In my opinion this marriage was almost dead prior to the violence becoming a real problem, and therefore the violence was not the root of the problem. Husband had shown pattern of extensive possessiveness, jealousy, etc., and *I believe violence was a result of the wife's eventual 'withdrawal'*.[1] By the time she came to me the wife clearly wanted nothing more to do with husband and already seemed to have come to terms emotionally with the marriage breakdown. The setting fire to the house episode seemed to horrify me more than the client! The other violence was no more or less than in many cases.

SOCIAL WORKERS

Factors

Case 5

[1] Cultural upbringing

The wife (twenty-five) *comes from unstable background*,[1] seems to *'latch on' to insecure aggressive*

68 Marital Violence

[2] Personality of man
[3] Interaction
[4] Role expectations of man
[5] Immaturity of man and woman
[6] Personality of woman

characters[2,3] Husband objects to wife leaving the house for any purpose. *Insists on her seeing to his every need.*[4] Arguments occur when she rebels. Commences with verbal abuse, progressing to him hitting her. Occurs about once a week. She presents as an unstable and dependent woman drawn to men of a domineering and aggressive character. *The husband (twenty) is even less mature than her,*[5] and resorts to violence *to assert his dominance in the family.*[4] He blackmails her into remaining with him by threats of going with other women and violence towards her by his friends. *Her dependence is shown by her frequent contact with me,*[6] indicating her plans to rebel against him, yet her reluctance to pursue this any further than her initial contact with me.

Case 6

[1] Personality of woman
[2] Cultural role expectations

The violence was brought about by frustration on the part of the husband when *wife persistently refused to clean the flat, provide regular meals and generally bestir herself.*[1,2] Both were unemployed and had lived together for eighteen months. Two children aged two and a half years and two months. Violence is a normal occurrence in this relationship, soon forgotten and considered to be part *of an ordinary way of life.*[2]

Case 7

[1] Immaturity of man and woman
[2] Housing
[3] Poverty
[4&5] Cultural upbringing and role expectations

The violence arose from a poor relationship aggravated *by the immaturity*[1] of the two people concerned, *the poor home conditions,*[2] social isolation, and *low financial state.*[3] *The wife experienced marital violence between her own parents and appeared to accept it as part of relationships far more than I did.*[4] *The husband appeared to see it as part of the normal way of controlling a wife.*[5]

Problems of explanation 69

Case 8

[1] Immaturity of man	There were frequent emotionally violent quarrels which culminated in the husband striking wife in the face. *He (twenty-eight) is immature*[1] *and has a hasty temper.*[2] *Wife (twenty-eight) is intelligent and independent and finds the closeness of marriage difficult.*[3] Therefore there are considerable problems of adjustment. She was illegitimate and didn't discover this until she was ten. Felt mother and step-father favoured other children. She did well at school but left and married at sixteen. At twenty left first husband. Consequently she had a great many painful experiences to work through and suffered from depression, but over years I've known her *she has matured and stabilized. The wife is the more intelligent and dominant partner.*[3] *Husband is attractive, sociable, but unreliable – spoilt by mother, also a gambler with criminal record.*[2] *Marriage has been stormy and stressful, during one period in which the assault took place.*[4] The violence obliterated her feelings of affection for him for quite a long time. Eventually she appeared able to accept the assault as part of his shortcomings, which she sees in a clear and detached manner. She has evidently decided that the positive aspects of the marriage outweigh the difficulties.
[2] Personality of man	
[3] Personality of woman	
[4] Interaction	

HEALTH VISITORS

Factors   Case 9

[1] Personality of woman

The violence was *due to maternal slovenliness and behaviour.*[1] The elder child was extra marital. The couple were married when the child was five years old. Mother was jealous because of love between child and husband. He was extremely fond of both children. She 'flew' from him after repeated violence and was away for one month. She completely disrupted the place where she was staying and eventually the husband left home with the children and went to live with his mother. The wife then went back to the home with her new boy-friend.

Case 10

[1] Personality of woman
[2] Personality of man
[3] Intellectual disparity

Husband has struck wife on numerous occasions and the wife has gone for him with a knife at least once. *She did provoke him by talking about other men*[1] *and by telling him that she had obtained a part-time job, which he had previously refused to allow her to have.*[2] *She is very discontented with him, especially his illiteracy.*[3] (Wife 19 – secretary. Husband 24 – council road-man.)

Case 11

[1] Immaturity of both
[2] Psychiatric disorder

In this case violence occurs most evenings. *Both are immature*[1] (Husband 23, Wife 21 – 1 child, another expected – cohabiting). Boy-friend is out most nights, coming in several hours late for meals. She has been very depressed ever since I've known her, exacerbated by present pregnancy and later by fact her boy-friend passed VD on to her during this pregnancy. *Because of her depression it is not difficult to see that there are problems on both sides in this relationship.*[2] She actually left for a women's refuge, but only stayed a very short while. She is very fond of the toddler and boy-friend threatens repeatedly to take him away from her. She despises him, but in reality he has provided her materially with a nicely furnished house and the child does not want for toys. However, her emotional needs are great and boy-friend gives her very little support.

Case 12

[1] Personality of woman

There are spasmodic bouts of violence approximately fortnightly – wife (twenty-eight) bruised,

Problems of explanation

² Inarticulateness
³ Cultural upbringing

black eyes, sometimes cut. *She is frightened of her partner (twenty-nine), at the same time enjoys playing the masochistic role.*¹ Threatens to leave him, but when positive alternatives are offered always turns them down. She is very loyal towards partner. *He sees himself as having to control wife – unable to find expression in words seems to do so in physical terms.*² Both partners in this liaison come from violent homes where parental violence was overt. *Their models of male/female role are probably taken from their parents.*³

DOCTORS

Factors

¹ Alcohol – man
² Personality of man
★ This is an example of ambiguous psychiatric terminology since it could be interpreted as referring to some deviance in the personality of the woman or, alternatively, may describe her reaction to her husband's violence

Case 13

Couple have been together nineteen years. No children. Wife came to me wanting to be off work for a week: 'anxiety-state'.★ She had been pulled by the hair and had bruises to arm and face. *He was drunk*¹ *and is a well-known psychopathic personality.*² I tried to persuade husband to come to see me but he would not. Wife later reported that he is 'very quiet' and remorseful and that a visit from me would only cause trouble.

Case 14

¹ Alcohol – man

Wife had been kicked and punched with fists. Injury to abdomen, bruising of the neck, thigh,

² Psycho-sexual problems
³ Illness of wife
⁴ Intellectual disparity

cheek, etc. She was admitted to hospital for three days. *Husband was drunk.*¹ *There had been frequent marital arguments about sex.*² She has had various illnesses since polio as a child. *Many admissions to hospital for abdominal symptoms, which undoubtedly put strain on marital behaviour.*³ There have been many episodes of violence related to alcohol, and his insistence on excessive and unusual sexual demands which were insisted upon in spite of recent surgery. Because of pain produced, patient grew to fear any advances made by husband. Divorce proceedings are now in progress. Clearly there was a *very unfortunate* marital set-up but it was aggravated greatly by the *male partner of rather lower intelligence*⁴ who, though able to accept his wife's mutilating operations, was unable to modify or adapt his behaviour towards her.

Case 15

¹ Intellectual disparity
² Cultural upbringing of both
³ Immaturity of wife

Wife, seventeen, married a year. Came to surgery with bruising of face, neck, and forearms. *There was an intellectual disparity between husband and wife – led to frustration on part of husband.*¹ *He had known violence in his own family as child. Her childhood too had been disturbed by parental disharmony.*² *She married at a young age to get away from the situation and made an immature choice which she has admitted.*³ The couple have recently divorced and she has remarried – no further trouble.

Case 16

¹ Alcohol – man
² Personality of woman
³ Psychiatric disorder of woman
⁴ Handicap of man

*Alcohol*¹ *and garrulous wife.*² There has been a long history of marital disharmony initiated during the *wife's prolonged post-natal depression*³ following birth of last child two years ago. Husband is *enuretic*⁴ – has become worse recently.

General comment on case-study material

It will be noticed that although all these short explanatory accounts contain mere fragments of information, they create an impression of masterful coherence. The essence of violent domestic relationships is often given in a nutshell. To practitioners that may not seem at all strange. For many, discussing and explaining their cases for other people is a part of everyday work. Yet if one reflects on this, it becomes apparent that the facility to give precise and accurate explanations for behaviour is a considerable intellectual achievement. Consider what is involved. First, an adequate amount of reliable information is necessary. Its acquisition is difficult because it depends on accurate observation of behaviour. Then one needs a capacity to weigh the accuracy of subjective retrospective accounts, often given by only one of the partners. This is extremely complicated where intimate partnerships and family relationships in general are concerned. One has to allow for the way information is communicated across the boundary between practitioner and couple, remembering the possibility that important information may have been withheld. Second, there are all the problems of judging the relevance of information and the difficulties of attaching meaning to it. Some of these have been neatly summarized by Marsden:

> 'Partial concealment, and the different meanings given to violent actions by the family themselves, can lead to confusion for outside observers, who may in any case disagree among themselves about the meaning of actions and appropriate responses.' (Marsden 1978: 123)

Furthermore, busy practitioners often have little opportunity to do more than gather snippets of information. They are also often forced to make snap judgements. It may well be that the busier they are, the more they need to be economical in their thinking, and the greater the tendency to over-simplify. The utility of 'shorthand' theory conflicts with the objectives of training institutions which, in general, seek to broaden and deepen practitioners' perspectives of the complexity of human behaviour.

Imprecise words such as 'deprived', 'immature', and 'unstable', recur particularly in the case studies of the social workers and health visitors. We also noticed in our interviews that these words seemed fashionable. They imply social deviance. Furthermore, violent behaviour was seen as symptomatic of something else which could not be directly confirmed. For example, the use of the word 'deprived' suggests an upbringing in emotional and material poverty, yet practitioners would rarely have had direct evidence of their clients' childhood. Likewise, the word 'immature' suggests the idea of arrested emotional development, and that the practitioner believes there are agreed norms of behaviour appropriate to particular age groups. We were left to speculate about the quality of evidence upon which such evaluations were based.

At first sight it may seem as if these practitioners are using a diagnostic model involving the following process: first, the identification of deviant or problematic behaviour; second, the acquisition and validation of information concerning the client's social circumstances and personal history; and third, the diagnostic application of theories to assist in the formulation of the practitioner's explanation for the client's behaviour. However, bearing in mind the difficulties that we have just outlined, it seems to us that the reality is often different. We think that the process of formulating an explanation usually takes the following form. It starts with the practitioner coming to the client with a 'toolbag' of shorthand theories. The problem behaviour of the client is identified. Then the practitioner proceeds to search, often quite cursorily, for evidence in the client's circumstances and history that will fit the favoured theories. In this way the practitioner's belief system, both in terms of morality and the utility of social theory, is constantly being confirmed and reinforced. This may have the effect of sustaining the practitioner's professional self-confidence.

Another point emerged from the case studies, although it is not illustrated in the examples above. In general, solicitors did not offer such full explanations as social workers and health visitors. They often confined themselves to saying that their client's marital relationship had deteriorated to the point of violence when it could not be tolerated any longer and required legal redress. While social workers, health visitors, and doctors normally tried to explain their clients'/patients' behaviour, we noted that some solicitors found it unfamiliar, telling us that they do not usually see the need to go into the whys and wherefores when a client seeks help. They simply act on instructions if the client has a legal entitlement. We have the impression that those occupations such as social workers and health visitors, which do not derive their authority to intervene directly from clients themselves, and whose practitioners are uncertain about their role, may feel a greater need to use morality or social theory as justification for doing so. In addition, it should be remembered that violent behaviour is often frightening and creates anxiety. After all, when people are made anxious and confused, it is natural enough that they should want to find a way of mastering their fear. Intellectual understanding may offer some comfort and reassurance in the form of rationalization.

Such differences suggest that each professional group is employing a different intellectual lens through which they perceive marital violence. If we are right in this observation, it ought to be followed up carefully, because the question arises how far cherished professional beliefs and mythologies distort the practitioners' perceptions of social realities. Some iconoclasm may be called for.

Discussion

Our study has been concerned with practitioners' use of explanations rather than with the validity of the explanations themselves. Nevertheless, alcohol, poverty, and psycho-sexual problems were mentioned so frequently by the practitioners in our research that we feel there is a very strong case for making detailed studies of the possible link between these factors and violence, particularly in the case of alcohol.

With regard to practitioners' use of explanations, certain propositions emerge from our evidence. First, it is not easy to identify the real causes of violence in marriage; second, busy practitioners tend to over-simplify; and third, there is a wide range of theory in use, often strangely blended with cultural stereotypes and morality.

May has studied the way previous generations viewed and explained family and marital violence and has shown the stereotyped images of domestic violence used by reformers and social workers of the Victorian and Edwardian eras. Our work indicates that many of these stereotypes are prevalent in the thinking of practitioners and academics today. Then, as now, the most common explanation was heavy drinking. Then, as now, poor housing and the emotionally impoverished cultural life of the poor, with its general roughness and violence, were considered important precipitating factors. Then, as now, social investigators were reporting the phenomenon of wives who take violence as a matter of course. Then, as now, references were being made to 'loud-mouthed viragos lacking domestic skills who often provoked their husbands' drunken assaults with their nagging tongues' (May 1978). There is nothing new in seeing domestic violence in interactionist terms. Furthermore, not only is recent concern about marital violence a 'rediscovery' of a problem that was a public anxiety a century ago, but, as our research shows, the old explanations for it circulate once again.

These points raise the question: What purposes are served by explanations manufactured from such an amalgam? Social workers, health visitors, and general practitioners, unlike most lawyers, believe that explanations are necessary in order to diagnose problems and decide treatment. They believe that the main elements of this approach are gathering evidence; defining marital violence as an abnormal problem; explaining it as a reaction to stress, or as a defect in the personalities concerned, or due to drink or drugs; and then, in the light of skills, knowledge, available resources, and agency function, choosing what treatment or help offers the best chance of cure or prevention. Although this is how many of these practitioners would explain their approach, as we have shown earlier, we think it is open to a different interpretation. Nevertheless the point that we wish to make here is that this approach, which may reassure practitioners by its familiarity, can be questioned on other grounds as well. Thus, one can argue that it is wrong to assume that practitioners occupy some kind of Archimedian point outside the patients' situation from which to make evaluations of their behaviour. Laing suggests that it is more realistic to see the practitioner as part of the very circumstances that are being diagnosed. He writes:

> 'What one sees as one looks into the situation changes as one hears the story. In a year's time as one has got to know the people and their situation a little, the story will have gone through a number of transformations. At a particular time one is inclined to define the situation in a particular way; this definition in turn changes the situation in ways we may never be able to define. People remember different things, put things together in different ways. This redefines the situation as changed by our (earlier) definition in the light of how it originally presented itself to us.' (Laing 1971:41)

The argument, therefore, is that a client's social circumstances may be altered by the very fact that the practitioner is defining, attaching meaning to, and explaining them. It is often difficult for the diagnostician to distinguish his part in the proceedings. We have several observations to make about this. First, few practitioners showed us that they were conscious of it when using the diagnostic/treatment model. Second, the kind of service that clients approach may well influence the way they present their problems. Third, it is probable that individual practitioners 'invent' explanations in order to convince themselves that marital violence is abnormal, when in fact it might not be (Kennedy 1981). One can argue that if they can convince themselves that it is 'abnormal' they may more easily hang on to the probably erroneous idea that the majority of marriages are happy and free not only from violence, but also from serious conflict.[5] Marsden, for example, has written:

> 'At a time when the use of violence in society is being challenged the discovery of the continued use of violence in the family conflicts with the idea that the home should be a source of peace and emotional support and renewal in a complex world.' (Marsden 1978)

There is a sense in which practitioners who believe that marital violence deviates from the imagined norm of happy marriage may be seen as perpetuating an ideology or social myth that serves to buttress faith in the institutions of marriage and the family. Skolnick has advanced such a view. She writes:

> 'At first glance it would seem that psychiatrists, social workers, marriage counsellors and other clinicians who help troubled families would be in a position to make unidealized assessments of family life. In fact, one might expect that coming into daily contact with family miseries, kept private from the rest of the world, would lead clinicians to exaggerate the dark side of family life. Paradoxically however, clinicians have contributed to the Utopian or sentimentalized model of the family: the clinicians' experience with troubled families seems to reinforce idealized conceptions of the "family" rather than challenge them. Thus the idealized model of the family remains the standard by which the "sick" families are judged.' (Skolnick 1973: 53)

Without wanting to weaken the general point that Skolnick makes, we should point out that her assertions rest on assumptions that, as far as we know, have not been tested. Remarkable though it may seem, as yet there are no research studies to establish what the norms of marital behaviour actually are. This means that everyone has to engage in a certain amount of guesswork. We think it reasonable to suggest that at any one time most marriages are probably regarded by their participants as fairly happy, although at some time or other they may experience unhappy episodes. For all that, the high incidence of divorce suggests that 'unhappy marriage', particularly amongst people in their late twenties and early thirties when most breakdowns occur, may be very prevalent. Nevertheless, assumptions of what the social norms are seem to us to be essentially subjective in the absence of empirical data. This means that assessments by professional 'experts' may be no more accurate than those made by laymen.

This line of thought leads us into the much wider field of social deviance. Goffman (1963), Becker (1963), Matza (1969), and many others have drawn attention to the way society differentiates between behaviour regarded as socially respectable and that considered deviant, morally inferior, and stigmatic (in the sense that individuals so labelled may feel that their identity or self-image is spoilt). Writers such as Robert A. Scott have examined the way professional 'experts' in social, medical and welfare services put people into moral categories (Scott 1970). Such practitioners can be conceived of as moral 'entrepreneurs who are at least implicitly (and often explicitly) generating the labels of what kinds of activities are respectable, normal, morally worthy, to be appreciated' (Ball 1970: 355), or the converse. When practitioners make moral judgements about their clients or patients, they are, in effect, treating them as if they are responsible in some way for the conditions in which they find themselves.

Much of the material presented in this chapter, and in the preceding one concerned with definitions, is open to interpretation of this kind. Furthermore, such judgements are made, as we have seen, not only in relation to the behaviour of the assailant but very often in relation to that of the victim as well. Sometimes judgements are specifically moral. More often, as we have seen, they are couched in technical, quasi-scientific terms. Nevertheless, if the underlying moral meaning is communicated to the client or patient this may merely sophisticate the form of stigmatization. It will not necessarily avoid 'spoiling' the client/patient's self-image. This may be one reason why women victims of marital violence are sometimes reported as feeling ashamed to tell practitioners about their partner's violence. It may also, of course, partly account for the fact that male assailants often try to keep their violence secret.

Denzin has suggested that the public disclosure of one's partner's deviancy may also involve a degree of betrayal and may hence be a way of shifting one's share of responsibility on to that person or even on to the person one informs. He argues that:

'The strategy for this action is clear, no moral responsibility can be placed on the betrayer, and the betrayed can now be shown to be morally incompetent, and hence no longer deserving or fit to be a member of the focal relationship. He becomes the perfect mark to be culled out by our agencies of social control. Of course once he has been shown to be morally unfit, all responsibility for maintaining the former relationship is removed from the betrayer. He or she is now free to enter into any other relationship. Thus having dispensed with a burdensome or troublesome partner, he can begin a new life in another moral order.' (Denzin 1970: 150)

Denzin's arguments, although they probably have some validity, should be viewed with caution. Those who have studied what women from refuges have to say about the development of violence in their marriages have observed that initially they usually seek help to enable them to continue the marriage rather than to escape from it. It is only when the violence persists, often over a period of many years, that they are driven to terminate the relationship (Dobash and Dobash 1980). Depressed and demoralized battered women have a tendency to blame themselves for the violence they have suffered, an observation that runs counter to the Denzin argument. Thus, we would suggest that his view is inaccurate or at any rate incomplete. Nevertheless, it is worth pointing out that his sociological interpretation of behaviour would seem to have much the same rationale as the psychoanalytic notion by which responsibility for behaviour may be unconsciously denied and projected on to another person, very often a partner or someone else with whom one has a close relationship.

Notes

1 The difficulties of mounting such studies would be legion: for example, sampling violent partnerships representatively; obtaining an adequate control group with which to compare them; and isolating the relevant variables.
2 Having drawn attention to the way academics, policy makers, and practitioners favour explanations associated with personality characteristics rather than social and cultural explanations, Dobash and Dobash write that: 'After such characteristics have been described, they are then usually compared in some implicit fashion with either the ideal of what a "normal" person (i.e. one who does not experience this problem) or family is like, or with some assumed, but unexplicated, behavioural norm. Through this form of analysis, the abnormal and deviant have been detached from the normal everyday lives of all of us, and from the historical and cultural legacy

of the patriarchal family. Thus, the logic of difference results in the conclusion that the problem of wifebeating arises from, or resides in, abnormal individuals and/or deviant relationships. Very comforting indeed.' (1979: 45)
3 This research is funded by the Department of the Environment.
4 The task of selecting the illustrations was difficult because we had 128 from which to choose. We have had to balance the need to be as representative as possible with a need not to be repetitive or take up too much space. We selected the most interesting typical ones, deciding that four of each would give a sufficiently representative spread.
5 It is estimated that 25 per cent of marriages will terminate in divorce on current trends. It is reasonable to assume that as many again will go through 'bad patches' but not end in divorce. The number of these marriages may well be much higher.

6
Questions of evidence

'It was a Sunday morning, that particular day, and he was attacking me with a sword. It was an ornamental thing, it had been given to our son actually, to hang on his bedroom wall. My husband was going to put that right through me. He was – oh, he was really mad that morning. I really thought he was going to kill me. And so I picked up the 'phone and called the police and they arrived. By which time he, when he saw them there, he completely changed. He was charming to them, you see, and it made it look as if I – they had a police woman there and she was very nice – but they could see that I was in the most terrible state. It was just awful and I was frantic and I was shaking. Then he lied about it all, and I was saying, "That's not true". The sergeant – it was a sergeant, said to me, "This is a respectable area and you stop behaving like a child". It was just dreadful it really was. When my solicitor wrote to my doctor, my doctor replied he knew nothing about it. I should have gone to the doctor. Only on three, I think, probably three occasions did I have any marks to show. He was very careful. He usually used his fists or he would do things like wind my arm round the banister and squeeze.'
(Housekeeper. Age: 38. Divorced. 1 child in her care. Length of marriage: 17 years)

Introduction

It is generally impossible for outsiders to learn the whole truth about violence inside a family. Often they cannot even find out whether violence which they suspect or others report to them has actually occurred. In this chapter we examine the way solicitors, social workers, health visitors, and general medical practitioners, faced with problems of this kind, try to acquire the evidence. To some extent their efforts can be understood as an attempt to get behind the boundary of family privacy. Their various approaches, and the standards of proof that they apply, are influenced by the way they define their tasks and responsibilities. They do not have a single standpoint. On the other hand, they are all outsiders and share certain assumptions about the appropriateness of enquiring into people's private lives, and when to accept at face value what people say. We have simply set out to describe and examine practitioners' general approach to the question of evidence in relation to marital violence and also in relation to non-accidental injury to children. Comparisons may be drawn between the two kinds of violence.

We have divided this chapter into three parts. In the first, we consider what health visitors, social workers, and GPs said they do when they suspect non-accidental injury to children. In the second, we examine what they said they do when suspecting marital violence and include the views of solicitors as well. In the third part we make some general observations and discuss some of the issues raised.

Part One

Proving non-accidental injury to children[1]

This is the aspect of family violence where policies have been most fully developed. The three occupations of social work, health visiting, and general medical practice can be regarded as three parts forming a single system whose task is to prevent, detect, and deal with parental violence to children. We consider evidence in this context first because it sometimes seemed to us to influence the practitioner's approach to evidence in cases of marital violence.

HEALTH VISITORS

Health visitors are the State's major child-care early-warning system. Jean Davies, a former vice-chairman of the Health Visitors' Association, summarizes their position in the following way:

'The health visitor visits the homes of all children under five years of age, and continues to visit whenever help and support are needed. She is thus in a unique position to detect early signs of injury and just as important, to recognize the conditions that could lead to it.' (Franklin 1975: 78)

Health visitors are constantly on the look-out for possible non-accidental injury to children. They are more conscious of this problem than of marital violence. There are set procedures to be followed, which reduce the individual health visitor's discretion.

In exploring the problem, we asked health visitors the following question:

'If a neighbour reported a parent being violent to a child what would you do?'

All but one said they would visit the family straight away and investigate. They disagreed about whether they should explain to the parents the reason for the visit. Thirty-three said they would not. A further six said they would only if they felt they had a sufficiently strong and trusting relationship with the parents. Ten, including some of the most experienced, said firmly that on principle they would always explain.

The question of whether or not to take parents into one's confidence when one suspects family violence runs throughout our data. We discuss its significance for practice and policy later. Davies indicates the dilemma:

'Should the parents be told of her suspicions? The health visitor can, under cover of normal routine visiting, observe without neighbours or relatives knowing that there is anything amiss. If she tells the parents of her suspicions she will almost certainly be refused admission to the house in the future. There can be no hard and fast rules, but the safety of the child must come first.' (Franklin 1975: 78)

We consider first the views of those who said that they would *not* explain the reason for their visit.

'I'd visit but not say why. I would try to establish rapport with them. If you see marks on the child ask the mother how they got there. If the story doesn't sound right and if it's the first time off ask her, "Are you sure you haven't got more to tell me?" You have to wrap these things up.'

Some told us that the policy was that they should examine the child physically whenever they were investigating a suspected case. This created difficulty for many, possibly compounded by their inclination not to explain the reason for their visit:

'It's terribly difficult. We're told to undress the child somehow, but that doesn't make for good relations with the family. I would rather find a pretext like, "He's due for a check-up in clinic – can you bring him in next week?"'

Health visitors have a marked reluctance to be authoritarian and to risk confrontation. Even those who said that they would inform parents that an allegation had been made, often qualified it by saying that they would only do so if they had an established relationship with the mother.

'If the mother didn't tell me, by some means or other I would have to examine the child. If necessary you have to come out with it [i.e. tell mother of report]. I try to start off by giving them the impression I'm on their side and don't believe a word of it, but the examination has to be done. They need someone to support them at these times.'

A few had no scruples about telling parents that they had received allegations and that it was their duty to investigate:

'I'd visit straight away to make sure the neighbour's statement was true. Women are so aware of baby-battering these days that I find it's all right to ask outright. They will admit so long as they know you're not out to get them into trouble and only want to help. Where they deny it I keep them under special observation until abuse is proven and give the mother support.'

Other issues raised by the question were how they would deal with the neighbours and whether they would identify their informant to the parents later. Several expressed concern that their future relationship with the parents could be jeopardized if it seemed that they were acting on false or malicious information. One pointed out: 'Neighbours can easily make a mountain out of a molehill. They might be being spiteful. They generally want to remain anonymous'. Another said that she usually 'points out to neighbours that they've got to be prepared to come forward to be a witness, otherwise it's only hearsay. You can't go and examine just on hearsay'. Another said it was her practice to 'go and see the neighbour to find out exactly what the complaint was' before seeing the family. Health visitors generally seemed reluctant to identify the source of their information even if they did confront the parents. One said dramatically: 'You would go into the family and find out what you can without involving the neighbour. Use the nebulous "someone". You lie in your teeth if they ask you if it was the neighbour'. To avoid situations like this, several said they would encourage the neighbour to inform the NSPCC whom they saw as having more authority to intervene and challenge the parents in such cases. On the other hand, one took the view that if the neighbour could be persuaded to be identified as the informant, it could make it easier for the health visitor to confront the parents with the allegation.

A number said that they would check with Social Services and/or the GP, sometimes to find out 'whether anything else was known', sometimes to put other workers 'on alert', and sometimes simply to share anxiety and the load of responsibility.

'Inform the Social Services Department. You must write it down for possible case conference. You have to cover yourself first. I would go in immediately and follow the set procedure. You must not be mealy-mouthed about it. You have to move.'

'Tell the GP first, and ask him for any information. I'd probably also inform the Nursing Officer in writing that I'd received an allegation. You have to play it by ear, you mustn't rush in blindly.'

It seems to be general practice for them to inform other services of their suspicions whether or not violence has been established, once they have visited the family.

'If I didn't get anything definite, I'd still write a report and tell the Nursing Officer. We pick each other's brains – another health visitor might know relatives of the family.'

'Even if I couldn't see evidence of violence, if the neighbour's complaint seemed solid enough, I would go ahead with the procedure, and I always inform the GP and the Social Services.'

SOCIAL WORKERS

Social workers were asked the same question as health visitors, namely:

'If a neighbour reported a parent being violent to a child what would you do?"

Whereas almost all health visitors said that they would visit the family straight away, the majority of social workers (thirty-four)[2] said that they would first try to find out what other agencies knew about the family. This was in line with agency policy which also requires them to inform their senior social worker and usually the specialist liaison officer. They are expected to make written reports of the allegation.

When visiting the family, social workers were more likely than health visitors to confront parents with the allegation, partly because they had less excuse for making a 'routine' visit unless the family was already known to them. Confrontation throws up problems which may be exacerbated by the policy of the social worker visiting with a specialist liaison officer.

> 'Often the CPV liaison officer and the social worker visit together. If they are not known to you, you have to explain who you are and why you are there. After that the interview takes off. They usually get angry so it's best to get in the door first. If you stay too long on the doorstep you won't get in. You have to be prepared to calm them down later.'

Others did not favour such forceful tactics. 'Would have to visit – see both parents – tell them a report had been received and ask for their side of the story.'

While most thought that they would have to confront the parents with the allegations, a few said that they might get another service, such as the NSPCC or the health visitor, to visit the family first. For example:

> 'If the neighbour's report was rather vague I would ask the neighbour to contact the NSPCC because we think their role is more acceptable. They have to act on any report whether malicious or not.'

> 'Although I would check it out and visit, I would probably get the health visitor to go in first if there was a younger child involved.'

Several favoured an oblique diplomatic approach: 'I'd visit as soon as possible. I'd start with a roundabout approach, talking about recent events to see if anything came up spontaneously and look for evidence of physical violence before saying anything about the report we'd received.'

GENERAL MEDICAL PRACTITIONERS

All doctors were asked:

> 'If you examined a child that had injuries that you suspected had been inflicted by the parents how would you respond?'

In answering this question it became clear that doctors often find it difficult to assess whether the injuries are accidental or deliberate. When they have doubts they usually turn to the health visitor and ask her to visit the home in order to get a second opinion. For example:

> 'I put the health visitors on to it and work through them because they usually know the family better. She can go into it and remove the child to hospital if necessary. GPs are curiously bad at recognizing child battering. Our orthopaedic specialist says that a fractured femur in a child under one year old is a battered child unless proved otherwise. I'm dubious about that. Accidents can and do happen. I'd rather be caught out by the odd rogue.'

> 'In the suspicious cases I give every parent the benefit of the doubt once. I say very little at the time to them but notify the health visitor to keep a close eye on the family, find out what she can and make a note of it.'

Thirty-nine said that they would either arrange for the child to be taken to the Children's Hospital for closer examination or, if it was less serious, ask a health visitor to visit the home and interview the parents. This seemed in line with the 'red book procedure'.[3] Typical replies were:

> 'I make detailed examination and enquiries of the parents. In ninety-nine cases out of a hundred I would refer the child for specialist assessment at the Children's Hospital to exclude previous fractures, bruises, etc. I perhaps over-react. I mobilize everyone. I'd ask the health visitor for a home assessment, inform the social worker and go over the child's medical notes to look out for previous suspect situations.'

> 'Do my best to confirm what happened by both medical examination and questioning of the parents. The nature and multiplicity of injuries gives it away quite often – just couldn't be accidental. Then I tackle the parents, and in severe cases threaten them with reporting to police. If she was not already involved, contact the social worker – they're jolly good.'

> 'If there is serious damage to the child both parents turn up. You get the impression of their panic. They make something up on the way round to see me. Their story usually isn't consistent. You get a feeling for the situation. Then write a letter or phone the Children's Hospital, and tell of your suspicion and suggest the child be admitted. They take it from there depending on the injuries – if necessary apply for a Place of Safety Order.'

Eight doctors seemed cautious about putting the procedure into full swing, unless the case was alarmingly serious.

> 'I saw a child with bruises recently and put on notes "beware of baby battering" but it seems a very happy baby so it's probably accidental. I think it's best not to challenge the parents outright but just to let them know tactfully that you're a bit suspicious.'

> 'I tend to play it a bit cool. I'd involve the health visitor and ask her to keep in touch with the family for me. She makes discreet enquiries and gives us feedback as to what we should do.'

> 'It's got completely out of proportion in the last twelve months. You are supposed to probe into everything. You can't clip your kids round the ears for being cheeky without risk of being a suspected child batterer. It's even happened to a colleague of mine, a health visitor, and she's a marvellous mum.'

Some mentioned that one problem of the procedure is that it presents them with a conflict of loyalties: i.e. how to help the child without getting the parents, their patients, into trouble:

> 'Doctors are not very keen on jumping in and causing problems or trouble for their patients, particularly if both parents are on your books. I prefer to ask the health visitor to call if I'm suspicious. She can then visit and if need be, involve the Social Services Department.'

> 'You've got to exert extreme care in dealing with the parents, so as not to provoke guilt or an excessive defensive reaction. I explain to patients that it is "normal" for children to get you to the end of your tether and that there is a temptation to violence. I try and indicate the possible dangers and explain that they need help and that it's available. I then ask the health visitor to visit and assess.'

Part Two

Proving marital violence

HEALTH VISITORS AND SOCIAL WORKERS

Both health visitors and social workers were asked:

> 'If a neighbour reported that there was violence between parents in one of the families for which you had responsibility, what would you do?'

Although there were certain differences of emphasis between the two occupational groups, the general range of answers was similar. Twenty-nine health visitors and twenty-five social workers were uncertain what they would do apart from making a routine visit if one was due, to see 'what came up' without alluding to the neighbour's report. Here are some typical answers:

'I'd go and see the family as a routine visit. Would see if the woman were to say anything. If she had a black eye I might cautiously see if she wanted to tell me about it, but I wouldn't ask straight out. If you do that she would probably only say she had bumped into a door. I'd pick up the bits as I go – you know gently work round to it, ask, "Difficulties with children? Well, how does father get on with them?" ' (Health visitor)

'I had a case like this reported by a minister. I visited and the husband was there. She had a black eye. I asked if she was all right. She said, "Yes". I asked, "What have you been doing?" – she said she walked into the door. I have visited since, but she hasn't admitted anything.' (Health visitor)

A number of practitioners said that they would do nothing at all unless help was specifically requested by the wife. 'I think it would be up to the woman to do something about it. I suppose they are sometimes frightened and it takes a while for them to tell you' (Social worker).

Risk to children was the main justification for making a special visit because a significant minority of health visitors and social workers seem to associate marital violence directly with the possibility of child abuse, as can be seen from the following:

'Marital violence isn't our business unless it affects the children.' (Health visitor)

'There's not much to do unless the children are under five. I would then do a routine visit on some excuse.' (Health visitor)

'If it is just between the parents we wouldn't be able to do anything.' (Social worker)

Comments like these seem to us to imply that the practitioner is redefining the problem of marital violence as one of potential child abuse. This may be another way by which marital violence and the woman's plight is relegated to the margins of the practitioners' concern and in some cases is in effect rendered invisible.

A further consequence of the child-care approach is that some practitioners thought that they should 'check out' the story with other services first:

> 'I would discuss the case with the GP first to see if he knew anything about the situation. I couldn't just go and present myself – I would need more justification for entry than that.' (Health visitor)

> 'I would ask around the office to see if anyone had up-to-date information about the family. I might well phone the health visitor if there were young children and might phone the school. But I wouldn't go and visit or ask the couple about it. After all, I've no legal right to interfere by going to see the parents about marital violence.' (Social worker)

Some, particularly social workers, said they would investigate the neighbour's story with the clear objective of building up information about the family even though a visit was not considered justified. For example, one social worker told us:

> 'I would try to draw out what I could from the neighbour and bear it in mind. This sort of information can help you fill out a picture of a family. If there is a puzzle with a missing piece – information about the marital violence might help. But of course you can't do anything on the hearsay of a neighbour. You can't go to the family and ask them questions about it.'

Answers such as these give the impression that many social workers and health visitors are prone to keep families under surveillance where they suspect marital violence. This is done not only by increased visiting, but also by alerting other services and sharing the suspicions with them, thus building up a dossier of information about the family even though the evidence may be unreliable.

GENERAL MEDICAL PRACTITIONERS

We explored the general practitioners' approach to the issue of evidence of marital violence by asking:

> 'If a woman came to surgery with injuries that you suspected were caused by violence from her partner how would you respond?'

Forty said that they would tactfully 'probe' to see if she wanted to talk about it.[4] Eight thought that there was little to do, either because they regarded it as an intrusion of privacy or because they saw no point in getting involved: 'I might say nothing at all. I'd leave the running to the patient, after all I can't do anything about it except advise'. 'Try and ignore it. Play it down. Attempt not to get involved in going to court.'

A number of those who said they would probably probe, mentioned the need to take note of the injuries in case they should later be asked to give evidence in court. The prospect of this seemed to worry them. Many said they were reluctant to do it but some said this was a consideration which made them more punctilious in 'probing' the nature of the evidence and recording it. One said: 'Quite often people come when they *want* you to record it and don't if they want to keep quiet about it.'

SOLICITORS

Since solicitors seldom have to deal directly with questions arising from non-accidental injury to children, we only consider their view of evidence in cases of marital violence leading to proceedings for injunctions and divorce. The basic question they face is how to acquire enough good evidence. We asked:

i) What standard of proof do you require in order to obtain an injunction?
ii) Does the question of establishing proof in such cases (i.e. obtaining injunctions) cause particular problems for you?'

Standard of proof

Twenty said that the victim's word alone was generally sufficient, provided that an exclusion order was not being sought. Only five said that they would always need definite corroborative evidence in the form of other witnesses or a doctor's report, although twenty said it was desirable. Some experienced solicitors said that it had recently become easier to obtain an injunction in the local courts. Thus one said:

'The standard of proof to obtain a divorce on the basis of intolerable behaviour has been coming down. The same is true for injunctions. Physical contact is no longer necessary. If allegations of threats are genuine that is usually enough. The wife's statement or affidavit is usually accepted.'

92 Marital Violence

Another remarked:

> 'I've done thousands of these cases. I know where the judges draw the line. It's in a different place today (1978) than two years ago. It used to be the case that judges would only order the husband out of the house if there was no other course of action and it was potentially dangerous and intolerable if he remained. They are less strict now. Years ago you couldn't rely on unsubstantiated evidence. Nowadays you don't need corroboration unless there is a challenge from the husband. In 99.9 per cent of cases the complainant's [wife] word is accepted without question.'

A number said that in their opinion, getting an injunction for non-molestation on a woman's[5] ex-parte application was almost automatic unless it was opposed by the husband or an exclusion order was being sought. We were told that in the latter case, because the man's property might be involved, judges rarely, if ever, granted ex-parte applications.

There were some solicitors who clearly thought that it was wrong to apply for injunctions on the strength of the woman's evidence alone:

> 'I do not believe that injunctions are necessary that often. Some solicitors rush off and get injunctions at the drop of a hat. They are abusing the power given them as well as the court. I always satisfy myself first that my client has really been subjected to physical violence – if possible with corroboration – or that she is in real danger.'

Another said:

> 'I always assume that the wife will exaggerate. You are sometimes told terrible things that aren't true. That's why I like corroboration – ideally visual evidence from a witness or doctor. Only if I'm satisfied that it was really serious would I go ahead without that sort of evidence.'

By contrast, there were solicitors who acted strictly on their clients' instructions, sometimes even where they thought the evidence was weak: 'There is never any problem if it's actual physical violence with substantiation. Mere threats may be more difficult to prove but I would have a go anyway for the sake of the client'.

Questions of evidence

Problems in obtaining evidence

Twenty-eight said that they did not normally experience evidence problems, since the word of the victim was usually sufficient. But those seeking corroboration encountered various difficulties:

(a) Mutual allegations

> 'It's difficult where there are mutual allegations of violence and where both parties allege the other is responsible. I have a case at the moment where neither husband nor wife seems to have any idea where the truth lies. The husband says his wife throws things about when there are disagreements, yet she goes and tells the neighbours that he is the one who has been throwing things so they think he is the violent one. It's impossible to get reliable evidence in that case.'

(b) Independent witnesses

Friends and neighbours who may have witnessed marital violence are often reluctant to give evidence: 'An injunction protects the wife but not the witnesses. They can be afraid of recriminations, and therefore not want to get involved'.

(c) Victim changes mind

This is such a common occurrence that we have written a separate chapter about it. It obviously creates difficulties for a solicitor who has prepared a case:

> 'You often find a client comes in in a state. You take instructions. Papers are prepared – affidavits, the lot. Then they calm down and have lost interest in a day or two. I had a case last week, a woman whom I judged to be over-reacting. I was right. Once she was off the boil she didn't want anything done.'

(d) Medical evidence

A number of solicitors mentioned various difficulties in obtaining medical evidence, including the reluctance of some GPs to provide it, delay in receiving reports and sometimes insufficient or inappropriate evidence in the medical report itself:

> 'Most doctors are reluctant to come to a court hearing. My first question to a doctor is, "Are you prepared to attend court?". Those

who have seen one or two broken noses are generally prepared to do so. One or two give reasonable reports. Others often write a report that is too prejudicial in favour of the client. Some of these tell the court what to do – "The husband in this case is a very bad man" – it's a waste of time for a doctor like that to give evidence.'

'It all depends on the doctor. I know of one Catholic doctor who is reluctant to give assistance because he is anxious to preserve the marriage.'

'Medical evidence can be difficult. Sometimes they are too slow in sending us letters. Then the report is too brief to be any use. Sometimes they are only provided on payment of a fee, but that's of secondary importance.'

'Can be a problem when psychiatric medical evidence is required. I find that judges often do not understand the doctor's diagnosis. Depression – mentioned in nearly all medical affidavits – without physical violence doesn't seem to appeal to judges.'

This last quote emphasizes one of the problems inherent in an interdisciplinary approach to marital violence. Each profession tends to give different weighting to different aspects of the problem. Here, the psychiatrist emphasizes the depression that women feel, whereas the judge is primarily concerned with proving whether physical violence has occurred.

Part Three

Discussion

All four occupations faced difficulties in acquiring reliable evidence of family violence, in both cases of suspected non-accidental injury to children and cases of marital violence. The main problems arise because violence usually occurs in private. Loyalty to each other or fear of the consequences of disclosure may incline family members to conceal it from outsiders. Consequently, if practitioners are to acquire evidence, they have in some way to overcome this defensive barrier.

A policy and procedure has developed to deal with this problem in the case of non-accidental injury to children, the key features of which are covert surveillance, quick response when suspicions are aroused, and close liaison between services. Minimizing the risk of physical harm to children is the primary consideration. Even so, it creates frightful dilemmas. If suspicion or allegation is misplaced the consequences for the family and children may be devastating: In *Re Cullimore (a minor)*, (*Times Law Report*, March 1976), Sir George Baker, former President of the Family Division, put the problem in a nutshell:

> 'The dilemma was that if the injuries were wrongly held to be non-accidental, the parents who were both twenty-five, could suffer unjustly and be held in hatred, odium, and contempt and pilloried in public while the child would be deprived of the loving care of parents and spend its formative years in an institution. If a diagnosis of "brittle bones" was made and that was wrong, the child was gravely at risk if allowed to continue living with brutal parents.'

Acting on the wrong evidence is unjust and acting on mere suspicion can demoralize parents and make it hard for them to remove the consequent stigma if they are eventually shown to be innocent.

We have acquired a good deal of evidence from practitioners to show that they are uneasy about these and other aspects of the policy concerning non-accidental injury to children. The policy is structurally determined by the problem of obtaining evidence, given the social norms against infringing family privacy. Martin points out that neighbours and relatives face similar dilemmas:

> 'Knowing that violence is occurring in a family poses tricky social problems for the neighbours. In England there is a fairly strong principle that what people do in their own homes is their affair, so that intervention can only be justified in exceptional situations. What is exceptional is a matter of social definition and the more uncertain, or even scared the neighbours may be, the more likely they are not to risk intervention.' (Martin 1978: 246)

Where marital violence occurs in families with small children, some health visitors and social workers seem inclined to follow the procedure for dealing with non-accidental injury on the assumption that the children may be at risk. These practitioners could be said to have extended this contentious policy to marital violence. On the other hand, we have little evidence to suggest that it applies where there are no children. Here the attitude seems to be that if the violence is between adults, outsiders should leave well alone unless help is sought.

Notes

1 Other terms used include 'concealed parental violence', 'child abuse', and, less often, 'battered babies'.
2 The remaining sixteen thought they would visit the family before contacting other agencies.
3 This refers to the book in which the local procedure agreed between services for dealing with cases of suspected non-accidental injury to children is laid out.
4 Many doctors said they found that women were often reluctant to explain reasons.
5 Several remarked that although rare, it would be more difficult for a man to get an injunction without corroboration. As one said, 'When it's a case of violence to a husband, in my experience they clear out. They say, "I'm not standing this" '.

7
Issues of privacy and confidentiality

Introduction

As we have seen, the problem of obtaining adequate evidence is closely involved with the issue of family privacy. This chapter examines the way practitioners view the notions of privacy and confidentiality when they deal with cases of suspected or confirmed marital violence, and discusses some implications.

Everyone feels that they have rights to privacy as individuals and within their marriages and families. They normally accept and respect similar rights for others. But the concept of privacy is difficult to define. Some writers point out that it is almost impossible to distinguish it satisfactorily from other concepts such as aloneness, intimacy, and confidentiality (MacCormick 1974). Indeed, the Younger Committee (1972) decided the term could not be defined adequately at all. In our study we wanted to find out how practitioners' notions of privacy might influence the flow of information about marital violence that they receive and transmit. We decided that it would be better simply to accept their interpretation of 'privacy' rather than to get bogged down in a fruitless search for precise meaning. By so doing, we might better understand some of the values associated with it.

Findings

In our feasibility study we discovered that social workers and health visitors in general were more worried about privacy and confidentiality than doctors. This was largely due to differences in the way they saw their role and how far they felt authorized to intervene in their clients'/patients' lives. We therefore explored the question of privacy more obliquely with doctors than the other three occupations which we consider first.

Solicitors, social workers and health visitors were asked:

'In dealing with marital problems are you ever worried that you are invading people's privacy?'

There are two aspects to this question: first, practitioners' views of privacy intrusion itself; second, the effect of these views on their approach to clients. *Table 7(1)* quantifies the replies to the question.

Table 7(1) *Worry about invading privacy*

	Solicitors (n = 50) %	Social workers (n = 50) %	Health visitors (n = 50) %
Yes	12	60	54
No	88	40	46

Some practitioners worried that clients can be drawn into saying too much about their private lives. Self-disclosure is irreversible:

'You are invading people's privacy more often than you realize. You have to learn when to stop confidences. Some are better not given. They can't be taken back. Some things are better not said.' (Health visitor)

'People often spill the beans when they are low but then regret it later.' (Social worker)

Practitioners often said that they could sense when they were approaching areas that the client or patient wished to keep private, as if there was an invisible but powerful boundary beyond which they ought not to go:

'To get to the bottom of their problem you have to ask personal, searching questions. If you think you've gone too far and are offending their sense of privacy, you should stop. One's personal feelers tell you how you are doing in a situation. Some mothers talk about sex for hours, others resent even talking about birth control. You have to tune into the context they find acceptable.' (Health visitor)

'I hope I've never probed. I'm aware when I'm getting into sensitive areas. Often you would like to know more to get a better picture of it, but you have to be patient. They won't tell you if they don't want you to know. People have been walking into doors for years.' (Health visitor)

Issues of privacy and confidentiality 99

Whether the boundary that people sense is drawn by the client or the practitioner is sometimes hard to tell:

> 'Privacy is a fairly constant problem. I try to take licence from the person or couple concerned. They give me the rope. I try to find their limits – how far they are prepared to go. Sometimes my reservations aren't founded, they are prepared to go further than I am.' (Social worker)

Some clients want the practitioner to start the conversation. One social worker said:

> 'I'm usually very hesitant about asking personal questions, but sometimes you sense that a person is longing to be asked a blunt question to unlock the block that prevents them from saying anything. It's not just how I feel, but how clients see me.'

Listening to people's secrets can be disturbing. Some practitioners said they had built up defences against this anxiety. For example, a solicitor specializing in matrimonial work remarked:

> 'You become fairly brutal. In human terms it's the price you pay. It wears you out – the most tiring work you can do – listening to almost insoluble matrimonial problems. After a while it makes you callous and insensitive to things like invading a person's privacy. Most of my clients really aren't precious – it all hangs out. They are not at all reticent.'

A social worker commented:

> 'Going into people's homes when they don't want you – as we do with court orders and so on – can be seen as invading people's privacy. All you can be is aware of it and compensate by understanding and sensitivity. I suppose you tend to become immune to anxiety about it. It's like a surgeon doing an operation – just another body you have to cut.'

A health visitor said: 'Perhaps I've become brash. If they can come out with it, whatever it is, it doesn't bother me'.

Privacy becomes a particularly complicated issue if a practitioner has been given information by one partner but not by the other. One health visitor explained:

> 'I don't like to hear the one talking about the other. Sometimes they tell you too much and then they are sorry about it afterwards. You

do feel you intrude into the couple's privacy when only *one* person comes and tells you things which perhaps they would not talk about to their partner. That's why I like to see them both together.'

Once information that is discreditable to the other marital partner has been revealed, it may become more difficult for a practitioner to remain accessible to the other partner. The disclosure of private information may be used as currency to 'buy' a practitioner's allegiance in the marital conflict. Furthermore, where a practitioner discovers evidence of violence by chance or by probing, he or she may adopt a partisan role that the client does not want. Even if the practitioner avoids this, the other partner, not having had the first say, may assume the practitioner has become prejudiced.

Solicitors encounter this problem less often because they represent or advise one party only and are usually cast in a partisan role. They are thus spared the tensions which arise from the need to balance the conflicting interests of both partners. This partly explains why privacy is less problematic for them. One solicitor remarked:

'Privacy is no problem because, if I am going into private matters, I am doing so by their invitation. They are privileged [he meant that the client is protected by legal privilege against the solicitor's disclosure to third parties] in what they choose to tell me. A client confides in a solicitor and knows that's confidential information. At the same time a client is made aware that unless he is frank with the solicitor it is not possible to deal adequately with the problem.'

Practitioners in other occupations also made the point that if clients volunteer information, intrusion is less likely to arise:

'If they seek your advice it's different from your having to seek information about them. Usually it's no problem because they've asked me to intervene.' (Social worker)

'It's all right usually because it comes from them to begin with. It comes out on the doorstep just as you are leaving. I'm only worried if I *have* to go and tackle someone.' (Health visitor)

The more practitioners see themselves as exercising control, the more they are worried about invading privacy. This dilemma is felt most acutely by social workers, particularly in relation to their child protection responsibilities, as can be seen from the following comments:

'What inhibits me is the thought, "Have I the right to go into these people's homes and start pushing into areas they might be reluctant to discuss?". It is easy to get out of what you ought to do as a responsible social worker and not to try to discuss difficult areas.'

'Privacy intrusion is just a fact of life in work with the local authority. I would say it's an issue in every case, how deeply involved you become in people's lives. Society, via legislation, seems to be saying we should play an ever-increasing role in the lives of families. This is the line that Directors of Social Services and local counsellors seem happy to accept.'

In child welfare cases, health visitors generally assume a more passive watching brief than social workers:

'I play it by ear. It depends what the problem is and how much they are prepared to tell. If they don't want to tell you, you don't probe further. I know where to draw the line. You can't demand to know every single detail.'

'I wouldn't directly ask them. They would approach me. If a mother had a dreadful black eye I would say, "My dear, whatever happened?", and if she wanted to, she'd tell me. I'm very careful not to interfere unless children are at risk.'

Doctors and privacy

Most doctors say they do not worry about their patients' privacy. This is because they feel bound by confidentiality, and because their patients generally initiate disclosure. In Chapter 6 we reported how doctors thought they would respond to a woman patient arriving at surgery with injuries suspected to have been caused by her partner's violence. Forty said they would probe tactfully; eight that they would not because they regarded it as an intrusion of privacy or did not wish to get involved. A number of those who thought they would probe, indicated how they would test the boundary of privacy:

'I'd say, "How did that happen?". If I get an obvious lie, I accept it. It would tell me more than if I was told the truth. If I know someone very well and she's got a nasty black eye and I comment on it – dead silence and then she burst into tears, I'd say, "Did you have a bit of a barney?", then I'd probably be told.'

'It's an old-fashioned technique. I sit and let the patient talk to me. Then I begin to probe and find the actual causes of the problems. I would ask outright if she didn't say.'

Many doctors suggested that it is common for victims of marital violence to try to conceal it, some to protect their husbands. Even so, most thought it was necessary to confirm the cause of injuries. The few who were reluctant to probe usually mentioned the patient's privacy and need to keep face:

> 'Tears can be almost an admission of relief. But if they put up a brave face I'd never break it down. I might make a note on their record that there is more to this than meets the eye and I would probably discuss it with my partners at our practice meeting.'

Confidentiality

From our preliminary work, it became clear that while some agencies adhere strictly to the principle of confidentiality, others make exceptions, particularly if they regard themselves as members of an inter-disciplinary team. There is much scope for misunderstanding here: clients can assume that what they have said is confidential to the individual practitioner, when the practitioner assumes that it is confidential to the team. Sometimes the practitioner may regard something as confidential when the client does not object to disclosure.

All practitioners were asked:

> 'Are there any situations involving *family* violence of any kind in which you would feel justified in passing on confidential information to another agency without the consent of your patient/client?'

Table 7(2) shows that solicitors differ markedly from social workers and health visitors in their response.

Table 7(2) *Passing on confidential information*

	Solicitors (n = 50) %	Social workers (n = 50) %	Health visitors (n = 50) %	GPs (n = 50) %
Would not pass on information without client's/patient's consent	26	10	6	16
Uncertain whether would	12	–	4	8
Would under certain circumstances	62	90	90	76

Many practitioners would disregard confidentiality when children are at risk. Social workers, health visitors, and GPs are all part of an established apparatus dealing with non-accidental injury to children. The policy encourages rapid informal communication between the services involved.[1] Not surprisingly, we received many comments such as:

> 'If children are at risk you have to. You can't worry about trimmings then.' (Health visitor)
>
> 'Oh yes, with battered children. Of overriding importance is the safety of the child.' (Doctor)
>
> 'In the case of children it's the safest and most expedient thing to do. It's now part of the established protocol. In the long term it may make families more defensive and suspicious of us.' (Social worker)

Some health visitors and doctors are cautious about passing on confidential information to law enforcement agencies such as the police or the NSPCC even though these services have child protection responsibilities. For example, one health visitor said: 'If a child was at risk I would always tell the doctor. It's more difficult when you go outside the medical profession and they don't understand the implications of confidentiality'.
Another remarked:

> 'To the GP yes, and to other health visitors. The NSPCC and social workers perhaps. To Child Guidance I might sketch a few details – possibly also the same for hospitals. But not for Probation. Definitely not to the police except at case conferences. Even there I hesitate about passing on confidential information.'

As solicitors are not part of the formal preventive child-care network, we asked:

> 'If it became apparent in dealing with a matrimonial case that a child was being subjected to violence what, if anything, would you do?'

Table 7(3) summarizes their replies.

Most felt bound to break confidence and inform the authorities. This is remarkable bearing in mind that lawyers may not disclose to the police evidence of felonies committed by their clients (Council of the Law Society 1974). One said: 'There *must* be some occasions if a child

Table 7(3) *What solicitor would do if child was victim of violence*

Solicitors (n = 50)	%
Contact other agencies regardless of client's consent	48
Could do nothing while they were clients	22
Other, including contact other spouse's solicitor	14
Don't know – hope it never happens	6
No response	10

is at risk, when you have to tell the police and damn the consequences'. Even so, virtually all said they would be reluctant to do so because it would infringe the privileged relationship with their client.[2] The argument against informing was put by one solicitor in the following way:

> 'I'd never do it. It's a rule of practice. As a solicitor you have to try and tackle problems like risk to children in terms other than disclosing confidence. Once you disclose professional confidences you are beginning to be judge and jury – informant too. So you have to stick by your client through thick and thin and do all you can to defuse the problem some other way.'

Some solicitors explained how they might try to safeguard the child:

> 'I'd put a lot of pressure on my client to do something about it. But I can't think of an occasion when I would deliberately set out to pass on information. I'd not shop my clients and report them to the social services department or the police. That would be totally and directly unprofessional. I would risk being struck off.'

Another said:

> 'I'd be sorely tempted to notify somebody, but I would be in great conflict because I value highly the confidentiality between solicitor and client. I would, of course, read the riot act – what good that would do I don't know. There's a limit to what else I could do. My hands would be very much tied. I could only inform the NSPCC or the other side [solicitor representing other spouse] if it were not in breach of confidence.'

Few practitioners felt that the risk to a victim of marital violence justified disclosure of confidential information. Indeed, many specifically excluded it, as the following typical comments show:

> 'Not unless children were being battered. They are not responsible like adults.' (Doctor)
>
> 'If children were involved I would pass on more freely than if it were marital violence simply because children are more defenceless.' (Social worker)
>
> 'In some cases where there is violence to children I definitely would. The whole CPV[3] system is set up so that it happens like that. But we haven't the same answers with marital violence.' (Health visitor)

Confidentiality and the primary health care team

Doctors and health visitors usually see themselves as part of a team within which it is generally accepted that confidential information about patients can be exchanged. We asked them whether they would normally inform each other when they encountered a case of marital violence. We wished to discover first, who they included in the team and how they drew the boundary around it; second, whether, in general, GPs differed from health visitors in how they did this; and third, how these factors influenced the flow of information about cases of marital violence between members of the team. *Table 7(4)* indicates the doctors' replies to the question: 'When you encounter a case of marital violence would you normally inform the health visitor?'.

Table 7(4) *Whether doctor would inform health visitor about marital violence (n = 50)*

	%
Usually	38
Only if she can do something	26
If children involved	26
Never	8
Not applicable, no health visitor	2

Health visitors usually see the membership of the health care team as comprising the GP, the Nursing Officer (District Nursing), and sometimes the local authority social worker. They were asked:

'When you encounter cases involving marital violence would you normally inform other members of the primary health care team about it?'

The answers are quantified in Table 7(5).

Table 7(5) *Willingness to report marital violence to other members of team (n = 50)*

(a) General practitioner	%
Always	76
Almost always	6
Occasionally	18

(b) Nursing officer (District nursing)	
If child at risk	38
Always	20
If serious	20
Never	22

(c) Local authority social worker	
Sometimes	76
Always	18
Never	4
No response	2

A comparison of *Tables 7(4)* and *7(5)* suggests that health visitors communicate in these circumstances more often than doctors. This may be simply because almost all the cases of marital violence they deal with involve children, whereas doctors will encounter cases amongst childless couples. Because some health visitors see social workers as part of the team, they are more likely than GPs to pass on information to them. Some doctors may not realize that a health visitor is liable to do this when they tell her about a case of marital violence. Others are clearly worried about the ethics of this:

'Especially if children are involved, it's essential to tell the health visitors and possibly the Social Services. You have to be very cautious and give only limited access. Medical records here are open to health visitors and ancillary workers. You have to be cautious especially if *both* partners are my patients. I still respect medical confidentiality. I certainly wouldn't discuss it in court unless ordered to by the judge – that has happened to me.'

Another commented:

'We are always passing on without the patient's consent – every GP has to. When any person is referred to another agency one should, in practice, get written consent to divulge information. The medical referral system relies on implicit consent of patients to pass information from one professional to another. Patients might not be aware of this. The medical system would break down if we couldn't do it. But the whole system is fraught with difficulties – there are far too many loopholes for confidential information to leak out.'

Discussion

Three questions are raised by this examination of privacy and marital violence: first, what does it tell us about the nature of privacy itself? Second, how might privacy influence the way marital violence comes to the attention of public services? Third, might privacy actually increase the likelihood of marital violence?

THE NATURE OF PRIVACY

Everyone we interviewed had a fairly firm idea what privacy meant. All saw it as being an important social value, probably a basic psychological need. Most differentiated between aspects of their clients' lives that they regarded as private and those that they did not. Most thought that they could sense when a client wanted to keep something private. Obvious though these observations may be, we felt they required closer examination in the light of recent writings on privacy.

Most academics discuss privacy in the context of individuals rather than couples, families, or larger groups. Therefore, we had to transpose ideas from the individual context and apply them to the couple. Ingham points out that 'there is virtually no empirical data on privacy' (Ingham 1978: 47), so that discussion is largely theoretical. This is almost bound to be the case, by definition, and will be a continuing obstacle to research.

Many philosophers take the view that privacy is the social mechanism that confers on individuals the freedom to determine the shape of their own lives, having something to do therefore with a sense of autonomy (Ingham 1978: 53). A right to privacy is based on the idea that there is a conventionally defined zone within which individuals should feel free to do what they like (Thomson 1975).

Reisman argues that acknowledging a person's privacy is tantamount to acknowledging and confirming a person's sense of self, since 'a self is at least in part a human being who regards his existence, his thought, his body, his actions as his own . . . the self requires the social rituals of privacy to exist' (Reisman 1976: 39). He goes on to argue that privacy is a basic precondition for regarding oneself as an entity capable of acquiring rights: 'Personal and property rights presuppose an individual with title to his existence – and privacy is the social ritual by which that title is conferred' (1976: 43–4). There is something appealing and persuasive in this view. It is also useful to apply the argument to domestic partnerships and family relationships as a whole. When we speak of a couple's private life, and of not wanting to intrude upon it, we are in effect acknowledging that their relationship has a distinctive identity and that the partners should be free to develop it.

This brings us to the relationship between privacy and intimacy in personal relationships. Fried (1970: 142) argues that 'privacy is the necessary context for relationships which we would hardly be human if we had to do without – the relationships of love, friendship and trust'.

He suggests that the intimacy of these relationships is brought about by the sharing of information about one's actions, beliefs, and emotions, 'which one does not share with all and which one has the right not to share with anyone. By conferring this right, privacy creates the moral capital which we spend in love and friendship'.

Even Reisman, who does not always agree with Fried, finds this analysis compelling. He points out that it goes some way to making jealousy understandable: 'If the value, indeed the very reality of my intimate relationship with you lies in your sharing with me what you don't share with others, then if you do share it with another, what I have is literally decreased in value and adulterated in substance' (1976: 32). This argument may explain why one partner may feel resentful when discovering that the other has disclosed to outsiders something regarded as private to the couple.

The knowledge that each has about the other, coupled with their power to withhold it from or communicate it to the outside world, gives both some kind of hold over the other. The power to disclose or withhold knowledge of oneself to the other is also an important part of the power structure in any relationship. Our research focuses primarily on the couple's relationship to the outside world and therefore we have not been able to examine privacy in the context of the relationship between marital partners. We think this would be a very fruitful area for further study. It might increase our understanding of the power balance in relationships, of the balance between intimacy and emotional distance, and of boundary control between the partners themselves and its relationship to identity and self-esteem.

Derlega and Chiakin (1977) suggest that we can best understand the nature of privacy by examining the ways in which the 'self-boundary' around an individual can be controlled. They argue that as long as individuals control what they choose to disclose about themselves to others, they can maintain privacy. Others, including Westin (1967) and Altman (1975), argue that the ability to keep personal information secret or to disclose it is vital if an individual is to maintain a sense of worth and personal independence.

The boundary around a partnership is affected when one or both of the partners has contact with an outsider. Control of this boundary may be exercised by the couple themselves and/or outsiders. A violent husband may frighten his wife into keeping knowledge of his violence secret. But at the same time the wife has the capacity to inform the outside world about it, and the consequent power to discredit or shame the husband. This can be a way of controlling the husband's violence. The possession of secret information by one partner about the other gives that partner power over its use. Goode (1971) suggests that physical force and its threat is used in all social systems as one of several 'sets of resources by which people can move others to serve their ends' and to control their behaviour. The other resources he suggests are economic power, prestige, friendship, and love, all of which contribute to the power structure of the system. By this line of reasoning one can argue that the power structure of the partnership itself will affect how partners regulate their joint boundary with the outside world. Into this will come a lot of other matters such as the degree of loyalty and affection they have for each other, the degree of economic dependence and the self-esteem that they derive from the partnership itself. It is hardly surprising that the weaker partner might feel the need to recruit allies and widen the audience, while the stronger may seek to prevent this. Thus, the way in which the power-balance of a partnership is managed may influence what information about it the partners choose to disclose to the outside world, how they do it, and whom they choose to tell.

There are many ways in which outsiders can penetrate partnership boundaries. What practitioners offer, coupled with the needs of their clients/patients, may induce disclosure of information. For example, you may have to convince people that you are a battered wife either to get into a refuge or to qualify for local authority housing under the Housing (Homeless Persons) Act 1977. To obtain a quick divorce under Section 1(2)(b) of the Matrimonial Causes Act 1973, you have to tell your solicitor and the court about domestic incidents that you might otherwise prefer to keep private. The price of help can be that one or both partners must give information about themselves to a wide range of persons and organizations and trust that it will be used wisely. Winning the trust of clients/patients so that they disclose this information, knowing when and how to ask the appropriate questions to elicit it, and recognizing possible clues about the nature of that information are all part of the range of skills that practitioners develop to gain access to private information. These skills are usually backed up by actual or implied promises of confidentiality and codes of ethics, which help practitioners to neutralize the defensive boundary of privacy.

The statutory powers of organizations such as the police and the social services to intervene and seek information can also be viewed as part of the armoury available to outsiders to breach and control partnership boundaries. This is not the place to discuss possible misuse or abuse of such powers. Suffice it to say that complicated power structures now exist to acquire information about marital and other family violence. In so far as this happens, the freedom of the partners themselves to regulate their boundary in general is reduced. That may have far-reaching consequences for the relationship itself. Once a boundary is broken it may be difficult to repair. Information once public can never be private again.

Socially deprived families are forced to seek help from a range of social support and social control agencies and often have to reveal a lot about themselves in the process. Middle-class and professional families, having more resources of their own, may avoid having to do so. Where marital violence is concerned, these agencies will acquire greater knowledge of its occurrence amongst poorer people.[4] In the process they will lose a measure of freedom in so far as retention of their privacy would have enhanced it.

HOW MIGHT IDEAS ABOUT PRIVACY INFLUENCE THE WAY MARITAL VIOLENCE COMES TO PUBLIC ATTENTION?

As we have seen, different services have different standards of confidentiality. Organizations such as the Samaritans and Women's Aid claim never in any circumstances to pass on information about clients. On the other hand, there are those services where it is more than probable that information about their clientele will be made public regardless of the original wishes of the informant. The police, with their capacity to institute criminal proceedings, are the obvious example. Between these two extremes fall services such as those provided by solicitors and doctors who, in general, would only waive confidentiality in unusual circumstances. Yet other services exercise fairly wide discretion whether to pass on private information without the consent of their clients. Good examples are those whose tasks contain elements of social control, such as provided by local authority social workers and health visitors.

Unpublished evidence from our divorce research[5] suggests that people with marital problems do consider the question of confidentiality before deciding which agency to go to. Some women are attracted to refuges because they offer a secrecy that prevents the husband from following them. People who are afraid that they will lose face by acknowledging that they have a marital problem go to agencies that can provide help in a 'private', acceptable manner. This was one reason why solicitors and doctors were favoured most. Some people still hesitate a long time before commencing divorce proceedings because of the public shame and loss of status they think it involves. Goffman's writings indicate the elaborate means by which individuals attempt to preserve their own face or role and those of others (Goffman 1956).

Because privacy protects intimacy and because intimacy is an aspiration normally expected to be satisfied in marriage, it is understandable that women, when first experiencing marital violence and wanting to continue their relationship, should turn, as the Dobashes (1981) suggest, to agencies such as doctors and marriage guidance counsellors who are believed to have strict rules about confidentiality. There is less risk of diluting the intimacy of the relationship by going to agencies like these than to those which are likely to give wider publicity, such as the police and the courts. On the other hand, some of those who regard themselves as the victims of injustice and unreasonable treatment want public sympathy and support and want to have their position acknowledged publicly. They may want their 'guilty' partner publicly challenged, exposed, and punished, even though they may not want to share that exposure.

We have found it helpful to think of two potentially contradictory forces at work affecting the flow of information about marital violence – one seeking to keep it private, the other trying to make it public. In studying the response of community services to marital violence, one is to some extent studying the dynamic interaction between these forces, often operating simultaneously and creating ambiguities and dilemmas for the people concerned, clientele and practitioners alike.

Most anxiety about intruding into privacy is felt by practitioners in services that have both a social support and social control function and where the distinction between the two is unclear. Local authority social workers display this most clearly when dealing with cases of suspected parental violence to children – are they in effect policing the family or offering them support and encouragement? Often in such cases it is not clear how far the family itself or society is authorizing the workers' intervention. It may be that society is evolving services that find it easier to gain access to information about the internal world of the family by appearing to offer social support when in reality the primary purpose is to provide social control. Here ambiguity of function becomes the device to neutralize the defensive boundary of privacy erected by the family itself. The price in terms of anxiety and role confusion for the social workers may be high.

MIGHT PRIVACY INCREASE THE LIKELIHOOD OF MARITAL VIOLENCE?

Barbara Laslett (1973) argues that privacy has emerged as a major feature of family life, both in the USA and the UK. Important changes in household composition, which began to occur about the end of the nineteenth century, brought this about (Laslett 1972: 125–57 and 205–35). Until then, other people usually shared the nuclear family's household. The middle classes normally had servants, and the working classes lodgers, relatives, and adult offspring. Shorter life expectancy, coupled with larger family size, also meant that married couples spent less time on their own in the household than they do now. One can argue that the increased privacy of modern times has two important consequences: a greater freedom from the control of others, and less social support. Privacy, by weakening social control, fosters the freedom to be more deviant. There are fewer people around in the household to see what happens when tensions between couples arise or to restrain violence. Thus victims are less easily protected and assailants less accountable and constrained by immediate social disapproval. This line of reasoning suggests that increased privacy, and the reduction in 'close living' in terms of housing densities and design, could have led to an increase in marital violence despite the lack of any firm historical evidence to prove it (Gelles 1978: 179).

Laslett's hypothesis may also explain why family violence has become a major social concern in recent decades. The demise of informal social controls and supports within the family may well have led to a general reaction within the community to replace them with external ones provided by formal organizations of various kinds. This may explain the rapid development of modern child protection provisions and current attempts to find effective ways of dealing with marital violence. Yet a weakness of external organizations is that they are not immediately at hand when dangerous situations arise. The social norm of privacy largely sees to that, preventing the victim's cry for help from being heard or restraining potential intervenors.[6] Then jeopardy becomes the price of privacy. The irony is that privacy contributes to, and reinforces, the intimacy and sense of solidarity in family life that society values, while it also nurtures and protects the very conditions in which conflict and violence develop.

Notes

1 Chapter 6 shows that some practitioners have considerable reservations about this policy, partly because it tends to override the principle of confidentiality and partly because the procedure is bounded by a secrecy that excludes parents.
2 See Samuels (1978). Samuels writes:
   'The client-lawyer relationship is special and unique. . . . Without the consent of the client the lawyer must not disclose to any other person or to a court relating to the affairs of the client. The law enforces and upholds this confidence and privilege as a fundamental and necessary constitutional protection and right in a free society. . . . The principle stands largely inviolate. It does not extend to the priest, doctor, social worker, conciliation officer, banker, accountant or journalist.'
3 Denotes 'concealed parental violence'. Other terms meaning the same thing include, 'non-accidental injury to children' and 'child abuse'.
4 This points to the danger of trying to estimate the incidence of marital violence on the basis of cases known to such agencies.

5 'The Circumstances of Families in Divorce Proceedings', University of Bristol, 1972–74. See Murch (1980).
6 One can equally argue that the improved legal status of women and the greater availability of community services to help them, as well as the modern disapproval of violence, might well have led to a reduction.

8
Ambivalence in victims and practitioners

'I had black eyes and split lips and things like that. I mean, he never broke any bones or anything like that. And in the morning, when he saw a black eye, he'd say, "How did you do that?". I think this is why I stayed with him so long, because I knew that he was sick. He just could not remember the next day, he couldn't even remember getting home, let alone doing any damage.'
(Housewife. Age: 37. Divorced. 2 children in her care. Length of marriage: 16 years)

Introduction

A number of victims, having approached services for help, later change their minds about it, often as arrangements are being made to help them. The police, in particular, have been quite bothered by it, mentioning it at a number of points in their evidence to the Select Committee on Violence in Marriage. For example, Chief Superintendent Dow of the Greater Manchester Police remarked:

'I suppose we tend to regard a lot of very minor assaults with caution. . . . We go to the scene then the woman backs out. A fortnight later we are called again because he (the husband) is doing the same thing again. You have to appreciate how a police officer feels when he or she goes to the same scene over and over again and the woman backs out.'

The police claim that withdrawal makes individual officers cautious about arresting and charging violent husbands. It has also affected their general prosecution policy. We were told that in Bristol it used to be the case that when an assailant had been charged, if a woman victim changed her mind and wanted to withdraw, the police acceded to her request and offered no evidence in court when the case was called.

This led to instances where the court felt the police had wasted the court's time and ordered the police authority to pay costs. Therefore the policy was changed. Now, the police obtain written and signed statements from the wife before the husband is charged. If she then changes her mind about giving evidence the onus is on her, rather than the police, to tell the court. Police Commanders whom we interviewed thought this a better policy, since it gives them less discretion about discontinuing prosecution and makes them less vulnerable to the criticism that they are failing to enforce the law.

Solicitors, too, frequently encounter women who change their minds after having instructed them to commence proceedings for an injunction or a divorce. Some suggested that this occurred in about a third of their cases. Of our sample of fifty local solicitors, only two claimed not to have experienced it. Some said that it happened so regularly that they regarded it as normal. The Law Society estimates the proportion of emergency legal aid certificates discharged or revoked on proceedings being discontinued to be 'in the region of 30 per cent' (Lord Chancellor's Office 1979).

Our interviews with workers from the local Bristol Women's Aid confirmed Pahl's (1977) findings that a number of women return from refuges to their husbands. One of the workers in a Bristol refuge called these 'moth and candle' situations, remarking: 'some wives just can't resist their men when they press them to go back even though they know he'll be violent again and that they'll be back to the refuge'. We were told that if conditions in the refuge were improved, and if there were better alternatives open to the women, fewer would be tempted back to a potentially violent husband.

In our research we sought to investigate practitioners' reactions to women who change their mind about seeking help and to discover how the practitioners explained or understood it. We have termed this problem 'client withdrawal'. We apply it to two rather different situations: first where a woman, having sought help on her own initiative, drops the matter before much can be done; second, where a practitioner hears about marital violence in the course of other work with the victim, advises her, and she fails to follow the advice. It should be borne in mind that there is room here for misunderstanding between practitioner and client/patient about when the task has been completed. For example, a woman may go to her solicitor for help as a gesture to make her husband believe that she is considering leaving him, in the hope that the husband's behaviour will improve. She may not make this clear to the solicitor, who may assume that she is instructing him for divorce. If her ploy works she may merely tell the solicitor that she has changed her mind about it.

Response to withdrawal

Seventeen of the forty-eight solicitors who had experienced this problem found it frustrating and irritating. It often coloured their overall approach:

> 'We're reluctant to do much because this happens so often. So many act on an immediate impulse which subsides when they are faced with the cold reality of separation from their husband.'

> 'If I suspect it's that sort of case I don't go for a quick injunction. It adds to one's sense of frustration. You may well have a highly distressed client, but all that could change in twenty-four hours. Why? Because of the understandable difficulty people have in making up their minds.'

> 'Why does it happen? To be completely cynical about it, most of those who chop and change their minds are not paying for it. They're legally aided.'

The prevalence of such views, understandable though they may be, creates a serious problem for the woman with a genuine need for a swift, protective response from the law. If the solicitor she consults is cynical and uninterested, there is a risk that he will be reluctant to take the necessary action and her safety will be jeopardized. One of the problems is that, as one lawyer said: 'You can't spot the non-runners. If a woman presents as a battered wife there is no way you can say, "I think she'll go back" '. His response was always to proceed on the basis that the woman means what she says. So far, the Law Society seems to adopt a similar policy in relation to the granting of emergency legal aid certificates for injunctions. Their Report comments:

> 'It is extremely difficult to identify the cases which might end in a reconciliation. Sometimes this happens where least expected, where there has been much violence and hardship. It has always been the Law Society's policy that the balance must always come down on the side of granting certificates where there has been violence. How much worse and more justified the criticism would be if serious harm occurred because of the lack of legal aid to obtain an injunction.' (Lord Chancellor's Office 1979)

Thirty-one solicitors accepted that women in these circumstances often change their minds. A few were puzzled that it happens so regularly, but most could see reasons for the woman's ambivalence:

> 'It happens regularly. Once an injunction is sought or a petition gets going they worry about their future – accommodation, income, kids, access. They wonder, "Am I still in love with him?". The law is such a quagmire – they feel anything can happen and what will husband's reaction be then? "Burn the home down, take away the kids, try to kill me?". He may threaten to do any of these things. Many of these wives feel on reflection that a certain world is therefore better than an uncertain world. Their lawyers need a lot of patience.'

Most of the lawyers said that in such circumstances their normal practice was to keep the file open and to wait a few months before sending a bill or claiming reimbursement from the legal aid fund.

If one assumes, and we do not, that people normally behave logically and rationally, ambivalence is not easy to understand. It was noticeable that those lawyers who had tried to understand ambivalence appeared the most patient and accepting. This point supports the argument of those who would like to see greater emphasis given to the study of the social and psychological aspects of family life in the training of family lawyers.

We encountered a similar mixture of irritation and acceptance from social workers and health visitors. If police officers and lawyers expressed rather more annoyance, it might be because they generally have more to do when a woman seeks their help, and they face the risk that their efforts will be nullified if she changes her mind. They also may be more vulnerable to criticism, for example from the courts, when action is suddenly and unexpectedly discontinued. Nevertheless, irritation that time and effort could be wasted featured in a number of the replies of social workers and health visitors:

> 'It's so frustrating when this sort of thing happens. I feel that in future cases I should not react too quickly to them, but wait and see first what happens before doing much.' (Health visitor)

> 'It makes you feel a right fool – when you've been running around making emergency arrangements for them. I don't do that any more.' (Health visitor)

> 'It seems to be a pattern in these women. Experience tells us to try and make sure it won't happen before we act to help them. You've

got to be quite sure they've made up their minds. It shouldn't affect our response to them but I think it does. We have to be cautious and not rush straight in to help. I know that might seem harsh to outsiders.' (Social worker)

Reasons for withdrawal

All practitioners were asked why they thought women so often changed their minds. Answers were often speculative, indicating puzzlement:

'I had one case where the woman came four times for a divorce. That's typical of many. I don't know whether she's really frightened of her husband. Does she love him, or is she afraid of the future on her own and for the future of the children? Is she downright manipulative?' (Solicitor)

The following comments illustrate what practitioners think are the common reasons for withdrawal. Many can be seen as reasons why women find it hard to leave violent husbands.

THE PROBLEM OF FINDING SOMEWHERE ELSE TO LIVE

'Very often they have nowhere else to go. No relatives nearby. She may think, "Why should I leave my home and the children's home?". There's lots of procedures to go through if they are to go to a refuge. Sometimes it's miles away. They have to sort out money before they leave. They have to start separation or divorce proceedings usually before they can be rehoused by the local authority. Sometimes they have to have obtained the custody of the children before the local authority will evict the husband. In fact it's surprising that so many women do get out because it's so difficult.' (Social worker)

'They often have more to gain by going back – roof over their head, someone to pay the bills – and feel most secure there. I hear this story again and again. Much more so than any complicated masochistic tendency.' (Doctor)

CONSIDERATION FOR CHILDREN

'They sometimes feel they're depriving the kids of their father, that if they leave, the children will miss their father. Some women feel it's worth putting up with a lot of shit for that.' (Social worker)

'I've a woman who has left several times but she always seems to leave a vital clue so that her husband will find her. She's genuinely frightened of her husband – I've seen her shaking. She's had a rotten life: divorced one husband; poor family ties. Anyone who cares about her, even if violent, is better than no-one. This husband is fond of her child and that seems to sway her.' (Health visitor)

CHANGING MIND AFTER CRISIS OR EPISODE IS OVER

'Often it happens at a crisis point and it just blows over. Once all is well again and the bout of violence is over they don't dwell on it or bother too much about it happening again.' (Health visitor)

'Some women are very volatile, so they react and then change their minds later. The media and all this publicity about battered wives encourages them to rush off to a lawyer. When they've calmed down they just want to go on leading their normal lives.' (Solicitor)

DEMORALIZED AND UNABLE TO COPE ALONE

'Being a victim of violence tends to erode your self-confidence. They become helpless and demoralized by the violence.' (Social worker)

'The women get so cowed, enmeshed in family routine, they lose their independence and the mental wherewithal and resilience to stand up to the man. I've recently had a case where the woman had nowhere else to go with the children and no energy. In theory it's easier for a woman to leave now but that's still often not the reality.' (Solicitor)

INTIMIDATION BY HUSBAND

'Some men make their life so difficult that the wife's rebellion is crushed, and she may be forced to decide that security with a bloody-minded husband is preferable to insecurity alone.' (Doctor)

'Sometimes the husband will ring up and say she doesn't want to go on with things. You wonder is he twisting her arm? All you can do is ask to speak to her or ask that she write to us.' (Solicitor)

STIGMA AND SENSE OF SHAME

'Some can't face the social embarrassment about leaving a husband who has beaten them up – they feel it reflects badly on them when explaining – they feel people will think they must have done something wrong for this to happen.' (Social worker)

'They don't want the stigma of being a battered wife, and don't want it to be public knowledge, so back they go and hope it will go away. I have a case like that at the moment and find it frustrating because I can't understand it. The wife says, "Give it another month and see how it goes". It's been going on like that a long time now.' (Health visitor)

BEGUILING HUSBANDS AND FORGIVING WIVES

'Some of these men seem to have a fantastic facility for saying they are sorry. The women often believe it, and so it goes on until the next time.' (Social worker)

'So often they say, "He's OK when he's sober". If he's only violent in bouts, and behaves OK between and he's a good father, they think on reflection that they can tolerate it.' (Doctor)

CONTINUING EMOTIONAL ATTACHMENT TO HUSBAND

'Sometimes it seems to be a case of can't live with each other and can't live without each other.' (Social worker)

'One should not forget that there can be a link between real hatred and real love. Very often a situation of deep passion manifests itself in violence. If a man is acting out of jealousy his violence may actually be saying, "I love you very much". These kinds of cases often lead to extreme repentance. The wife loves the man and is prepared to accept it.' (Solicitor)

WOMAN NEEDS STIMULUS OF VIOLENCE OR NEEDS TO PROVOKE IT[1]

'It may be rare, but I suppose some women tolerate, even like, brutal men. I think they must quite enjoy it really. In some extreme personalities they almost need it. They only seem able to feel fully alive when their emotions are fully stretched. Merely parting from their partner leaves them feeling empty and doesn't solve anything.' (Doctor)

'Some women deserve it or provoke it – they flirt a bit. The husband's response is an old-fashioned cuff around the ears – like police used to do with kids – don't think it does her a lot of harm. Keeps her in line and she knows it – that's why she stays.' (Doctor)

VIOLENCE ITSELF PROVIDES SOME KIND OF EMOTIONAL SECURITY

'A percentage of women expect to be beaten and invite it because it demonstrates their husbands feel something for them. They don't feel adequate to cope alone – it's better to have a husband, even if he belts you, at least you are getting attention.' (Health visitor)

'I think some women get a kind of reassurance living in a very physical atmosphere. Violence is preferable to cold indifference, only when the attacks get very brutal or when neighbours, friends or even older children start telling them they shouldn't put up with it will they bring themselves to a solicitor. Some kind of gesture to their friends as much as their husband – and then they don't go through with it.' (Solicitor)

AIRING THE PROBLEM IS ENOUGH

'Coming to someone to talk about it and discuss it can make it tolerable.' (Health visitor)

'Sometimes they are just trying to find a solution to the violent behaviour – they can only think of seeing a solicitor. They want the violence to stop, not the marriage to end. After the injunction they say they don't want anything else. It might alleviate the problem in the short term.' (Solicitor)

SYMBOLIC GESTURE

'Some women seem to be saying, "I want you to tell that Judge and I want the Judge to put the fear of god into my husband". I think that's the psychology of it . . . I'm not saying they are not genuinely disturbed, but expressly or impliedly they are using the system for a good telling off. Solicitors, judges, social workers are all pawns in the game.' (Solicitor)

'In some cases where they go back some good has been done. Just by coming to see us and showing the husband she's serious she demonstrates a modicum of independence. After that the husband might realize he can't do just as he pleases with her.' (Solicitor)

RECONCILIATION CAN BE GENUINE

'Eighteen months ago I had a very bad case. The wife had a broken arm. The husband had a drink problem. Violence was almost a nightly occurrence. I prepared a petition and said we should apply for an injunction since it was the clearest case of severe violence we've ever had. She went away and 'phoned me the next day and said, "I don't want to go ahead". I kept the file open and wrote to her six months later to see how she was. It turned out she was very happy and the violence seemed to have stopped.' (Solicitor)

THE SERVICE OFFERED IS NOT WHAT CLIENT WANTS

'They discontinue because you can't help. They don't get what they want from you. It's too threatening when you dig up what's going on.' (Doctor)

'People withdraw when you try to examine the situation in a neutral way. That threatens their interpretation of the problem. You'll get a woman saying, "My husband's mad: I want you to get him locked up". If you then say, "Well, perhaps he's not mad, let's look at what's happening between you" – that's when they back away.' (Social worker)

Discussion

Client withdrawal happens fairly often and it sometimes makes practitioners cautious about responding. A woman's safety may consequently be at risk. Furthermore, it seems likely that if she encounters a sceptical attitude, the woman may be demoralized into thinking that her plight is not being taken seriously. One can understand why practitioners are cautious, but that need not involve rejection, provided they understand the part that ambivalence plays in marital relationships and the bonds that hold people together, even in the most difficult and dangerous circumstances.[2] Another aspect is that the woman's uncertainty in these circumstances may feed and reinforce the more general uncertainties about role in dealing with marital problems that some practitioners experience, particularly social workers, health visitors, and general practitioners. Furthermore, some women may sense that the practitioner expects them to withdraw which may even serve to encourage it. Overall it could be that the problem of client withdrawal reflects a wider societal ambivalence about marital violence. In this way it is rather similar to, and indeed may be confused with, the ambivalence associated with privacy intrusion examined in the previous chapter.

Nevertheless, in our opinion, the question of withdrawal is central to the whole problem of marital violence; not least because it is often seen as an excuse for inaction. Those interviewed talked more freely about withdrawal than about privacy, probably because they had more facts and anecdotes to support their opinions. Government, through record-keeping and agencies such as the police, health, and education services, constantly infringe people's privacy without their consent – indeed often without their knowledge. But what is particularly noticeable about marital violence is the reluctance to interfere even when asked. This attitude seems to stem largely from the real or apparent ambivalence of the victims of violence towards their situation and its resolution when, for instance, they return home or withdraw from agency help or legal action.

Against this background, it is important to stress the severe practical difficulties of taking unequivocal action – and that, in spite of these, many women do not withdraw but proceed with it. Furthermore, there seems to be little evidence of conscious ambivalence about the violent behaviour – they want that to stop. Their problem is how to accomplish this without total upheaval and loss of security. These women often seek help at a time of great stress, when they feel they have reached breaking point and urgently need protection and/or separation from the man. In this state they may initiate legal proceedings, demand refuge or re-housing. Once the immediate crisis is over, their needs and priorities may change; the pressing everyday needs for clean clothes, housekeeping money, one's own home, or the need to keep the family together for the children's sake reassert themselves. At this point many women return home. As we have seen, by so doing, they may alienate those who have sympathized and offered help.

The Dobashes (1980: 144–60) have shown in their study of women from refuges how many women made a number of attempts to leave home and escape the violence as the couple's relationship deteriorated. Practitioners may fail to appreciate the complex feelings the woman may be experiencing. They may be under the misconception that by returning home the woman is implying that the help and intervention were not necessary. Take the analogy of a serious car accident. The immediate need is for medical attention. It does not matter about the car, the business you were engaged on when the accident happened, your work or money problems. All you want is to survive. Afterwards, as you recover, other problems surface: you may feel impatient about the treatment or discharge yourself from hospital against medical advice to attend to urgent business matters, to start earning again. This does not mean that the doctor's emergency work was unnecessary. The later state does not invalidate the former need.

Perhaps it would be better if agencies could direct their attention to the earlier straightforward need in such a way that it does not involve the victim in hard-line action and the consequent need for a U-turn. We already have adequate legislation to deal with complete separation. The Domestic Violence and Matrimonial Proceedings Act 1976 helps by making it possible to institute injunction proceedings without assuming that a divorce will follow. This is a legal acknowledgement that wanting the violence to end is not necessarily the same as wanting the marriage to end, a point made to us by a number of solicitors. What is needed are practices and policies that recognize that there is a need for help – and often urgent help – before decisions about divorce and/or criminal prosecution are taken. In theory, the 1976 Act adopts this approach, but in practice, as soon as the woman leaves the home the question of re-housing arises, and many Councils will not take action until there is an official separation.

If agencies/practitioners could concentrate their help on the less ambivalent area of the situation – the need to stop the violence – it could conceivably minimize the stresses the victims experience and the uncertainties of those who try to help them. If there were alternative methods of dealing with the problem that fell short of splitting the family permanently and putting the woman and children into a difficult, insecure, even homeless situation, practitioners would perhaps feel more confident about so-called interfering. This could be particularly important for health visitors and social workers whose training and statutory responsibilities make them very aware of risks to children.

Notes

1 These quotations could as easily have been incorporated in Chapter 5, since they support the view that violence is due to personality factors.
2 This may have implications for training.

9
'Ignorance of the law is no excuse'

Introduction

Victims of marital violence have diverse social, medical, and legal needs. An approach to a particular service implies that they have defined their needs and selected the help they see as most appropriate. However, domiciliary services, such as those provided by health visitors and social workers, are more likely to discover victims who have not yet distinguished the nature of their needs. It may therefore fall to these practitioners to work this out with the victim.

Knowledge is one of the fundamental resources that determines a practitioner's response to a problem. We illustrate this point here by examining legal knowledge. Yet we could have chosen to investigate practitioners' understanding of other important areas, for example, people's psychological or social welfare needs. An advantage of investigating their state of legal knowledge was that the fundamentals of the substantive law are relatively unambiguous. Moreover, practitioners generally have available to them reliable sources of information in statutes, practitioners' guides and case law, so they can check whether they are right. Thus law is one of those areas of knowledge about which a practitioner can become fairly certain. Yet our preliminary work suggested that some practitioners' understanding of legal remedies was weak, although it is clearly a very important subject in dealing with marital violence.

Before presenting our findings we summarize briefly the main legal remedies available to victims. They fall into two categories: criminal and civil.[1]

CRIMINAL LAW

In the most extreme cases, the police prosecute under common law for murder, attempted murder, and manslaughter. Prosecution in most other cases can be initiated under the following sections of the

Offences Against the Person Act 1861:

S.18 – causing grievous bodily harm or wounding with intent to cause grievous bodily harm;
S.20 – wounding or inflicting grievous bodily harm;
S.42 – common assault;
S.47 – assault occasioning actual bodily harm.

In the case of Section 42, it is normally left to the person assaulted to institute proceedings. We drew attention in Chapter 2 to the relatively low proportion of prosecutions arising from incidents of domestic violence reported to the police.

Much criticism has been made of the police response to marital violence. In their evidence to the Parliamentary Select Committee on Violence in Marriage, a number of Women's Aid groups said that often, where asssault takes place within a person's home, the police are reluctant to intervene and commence criminal prosecution, sometimes even when the assault is serious. It has been claimed that the police apply a double standard whereby they are more likely to prosecute cases of assault committed in a public place than in the privacy of a person's house. There is ambiguity about whether this so-called double standard rests on a distinction being made between the private/public *location* of the offence, or on a distinction between its marital/non-marital *character*.

The police, in their evidence to the Select Committee, did not entirely refute these allegations; rather, they sought to explain them. They pointed to the difficulty they sometimes have in establishing proof in such cases: often they arrive on the scene after the events complained of have taken place. There may be no physical evidence in the form of bruising or wounds. Each party may make allegations against the other (Report from the Select Committee on Violence in Marriage 1975). Many women are reported to be reluctant to give evidence against their partners in court, sometimes wishing to withdraw statements given earlier to the police. The police said that prosecution may sometimes be unhelpful and may exacerbate strained marital and family relationships. They said that quite often the mere arrival of a police officer at a domestic incident is sufficient to calm the atmosphere and deter future assault.[2]

Women whose partners are prosecuted under the criminal law now have an opportunity to apply for compensation for their injuries. In announcing a revision of the Criminal Injuries Compensation Scheme in July 1979, the Government extended the scheme to cases where 'victim and offender live together as members of the same family'. This came into effect on 1 October 1979, on an experimental basis. Certain safeguards were included to guard against abuse. Compensation will normally only be awarded where:

1 The offender has been prosecuted in connection with the offence.
2 The injuries justify compensation of at least £500.
3 The board is satisfied that the offender will not benefit from the award.
4 In the case of a minor the award is in the child's interest.[3,4]

CIVIL LAW

In civil law a woman may apply for an injunction in the County Court, either under the Domestic Violence and Matrimonial Proceedings Act 1976, or in the course of divorce. Since 1979 the woman may also proceed in the Magistrates' Court under the Matrimonial Proceedings Magistrate's Courts Act 1978. The distinctive feature of the 1976 Act was that it was no longer necessary for a woman seeking an injunction to file a petition for divorce. It also made it possible for cohabitees to seek injunctions against their partners. Basically there are two types of injunction used in such proceedings: first, a non-molestation injunction restraining the other party from further violence, and second (a less common practice), one to exclude the assailant from the matrimonial home. Alternatively, the court can accept an undertaking from the offender that he will not molest his partner. Powers of arrest can be attached, to be implemented if the offender is in breach of the injunction. In cases where no power of arrest is attached, the sanction open to the court for non-compliance with the injunction is punishment for contempt. The offender may be imprisoned until the court is satisfied that the contempt has been purged. The weakness of this procedure is that it has to be triggered by the victim informing the court that her husband is in breach of the injunction. She may well be too frightened to do so. Moreover, Parker (1981) has argued that the developing case law concerning these two Acts shows that the courts have given them a restrictive interpretation.

The final remedy available to married victims is divorce. As can be seen in Chapter 8, the wife who changes her mind about leaving home or bringing a prosecution against her husband may well be reluctant to set the machinery of divorce in motion. As Baroness Phillips said in the House of Lords in 1976: 'At the time of probably having been beaten, assaulted, and thrown out of the house, bruised and frightened, the last thing a woman wants to do is start the complications of a divorce or separation proceedings' (Hansard 1976). We should remember that wanting one's husband restrained from violence may be quite different from wanting to live apart and, again, quite different from wanting divorce, a permanent legal termination of the relationship. Furthermore, a number of 'marital assaults' take place after divorce, sometimes arising from custody and access problems, sometimes over arguments about division of property.

At the time we did our field-work, the provisions of the Housing (Homeless Persons) Act 1977 had only just been brought into force. As our feasibility study had indicated that practitioners would not be conversant with the Act, we did not ask a specific question about it.[5,6]

Findings

SOCIAL WORKERS AND HEALTH VISITORS

Social workers and health visitors were asked:

> 'In relation to marital violence in particular, do you know what legal remedies are open to victims of marital violence?'

We were inviting practitioners to assess the adequacy of their own knowledge. We were not in a position to test and evaluate it objectively. Their answers are quantified in *Table 9(1)*.

Table 9(1) *Knowledge of the law*

	Social workers (n = 50) %	Health visitors (n = 50) %
Well informed	26	4
A little knowledge	68	28
No knowledge – would refer elsewhere	4	68
No response	2	–

Table 9(1) shows that health visitors are more diffident about the state of their knowledge of legal remedies than social workers. Neither occupation was confident and some practitioners clearly thought that they had no need to know the law:

'It's not our job – I keep out of it.' (Health visitor)
'We can't be practitioners on everything.' (Health visitor)
'It's not my role to know about legal issues.' (Health visitor)
'My knowledge is only at a fairly generalized level.' (Social worker)
'I don't feel qualified.' (Social worker)
'Better to get to a solicitor in case I get things wrong.' (Social worker)

We noticed that of those who felt they were well informed, many were vague about injunctions and none mentioned the power of arrest provision. Many of those who admitted to having only hazy knowledge were unhappy about it and often said they should know more. As one social worker said: 'The whole aspect of the law in the course was minimal – there should have been more. I wouldn't say we were trained – I feel even now I'm not qualified.'

As far as health visitors are concerned, it would be reasonable to argue that in a health-oriented service, knowledge of the law is of secondary importance. Nevertheless, health visitors were shaky in their knowledge of the law. Only thirteen said that if they encountered a case of marital violence with obvious legal needs, they would refer the victim to solicitors, law centres, Citizens' Advice Bureaux, or the Bristol Women's Aid. Four said they would refer to social workers and a few mentioned the police. One of these thought that the police might be useful for surveillance, but most were of the opinion that the police would not want to be involved in domestic matters.

By contrast, thirty-four social workers said they would recommend a solicitor. This touches on a point that we will consider more fully later, namely that social workers have a more positive view of the legal profession than health visitors. Only two social workers mentioned the police. Some social workers said that if they felt out of their depth when encountering a client's legal problem they would seek advice and information from colleagues, either other social workers or the solicitors working in the Local Authority legal section.

VIGNETTE TEST

Another way we investigated practitioners' knowledge of the law was by asking how they might deal with a number of situations of marital violence that we posed in the form of brief vignettes. By themselves these were not an adequate test of practitioners' knowledge, since they merely stated a problem to which there might have been a number of possible responses, social, medical and legal. Nevertheless, in our opinion, they confirmed these practitioners' general reluctance to consider and become involved with legal issues. Of course it is possible to argue that in these situations the law does not provide an adequate solution. We are not suggesting that the law is omnicompetent, but rather that practitioners working in non-legal services ought to be mindful of the possible legal options.

Health visitors

The first vignette question asked of health visitors was:

> 'A battered wife arrives at the clinic with her children. She has left her husband and has nowhere to go. What kind of help might you give her?'

The majority response was to give first priority to finding accommodation, often by referral to the Social Services Department.[7] Only three of the fifty health visitors mentioned that legal help would also be appropriate or necessary, and each of these said they would not have attempted to offer the legal advice themselves.

The second vignette was:

> 'You are approached by a wife from a marriage where there is a long history of marital violence. In recent weeks the violence has got worse and she is now frightened for her life. What help could you offer her?'

Only sixteen health visitors mentioned recourse to the law, seven of whom said they would refer to solicitors and two to social workers on the basis that 'social workers know more about the law and are therefore better equipped to cope'.

The third vignette was:

> 'When making a routine visit to a young mother she tells you that her husband can be violent and knocks her about. What would you do?'

Most of the health visitors mentioned a whole range of medical and social help. Only two mentioned recourse to law, one of whom suggested going to the police.

Social workers

Like health visitors, the social workers were asked to respond to the first two of the vignettes. As to the first, nine social workers felt the woman needed legal help and should see a solicitor. Three said an injunction would be appropriate so that the husband could be removed from the matrimonial home quickly, though one added: 'Injunctions don't always work – men don't take much notice of them'. Another said that she would suggest that, 'The husband moves out of the house so the wife and kids can return – there's no need to go to court'. Interestingly, two said that the woman should see her general practitioner so that he could record any evidence of the violence for future court proceedings.

In answer to the second vignette, ninteeen said they would send the wife to a solicitor, seven specified that this would be for the purpose of obtaining an injunction. Three said they would alert the police, one said erroneously that this would be in order to obtain an injunction. Three felt that separation, divorce, and child custody should be considered. One mentioned that the refuge had a good legal advice service to offer.

The third social worker vignette was:

'You are supervising two children in a family under Child Protection legislation. While dealing with other problems it emerges that there is some violence between the parents. How would you respond?'

The majority of answers reflected the social workers' concern about the effect that violence between the parents might have on the children, and most elected to help by offering counselling. Only one mentioned referral to a solicitor. Another remarked: 'I would tell about the legal side and the powers we have to take the children away'.

The evidence from these vignette questions supports our general finding that health visitors and social workers tend to consider other options before legal remedies, and that their knowledge of the law and legal services is weak. Given the peripatetic nature of their work we think they must be losing many opportunities to acquaint victims with a rudimentary understanding of their legal entitlements and with the knowledge of how to obtain them. This has implications for training.

GENERAL MEDICAL PRACTITIONERS

Because general practitioners do not have the roving commission of social workers and health visitors, and because patients were not particularly likely to seek legal advice from them, we did not ask specifically about their legal knowledge. However, references to the law emerged from the answers to the following vignette question:

> 'You are approached by a wife from a marriage where there is a long history of marital violence. In recent weeks the violence has grown worse and she is now frightened for her life. What help could you offer her?'

General practitioners were more inclined than social workers and health visitors to acknowledge the legal aspects of this problem, thirty-three doing so compared with twenty-eight social workers and sixteen health visitors who were asked the same question.

Twenty-four thought the woman should see a solicitor. One said a solicitor would be appropriate only if he thought the marriage had 'had it'. Eleven said the police should be informed, three of whom thought the police would offer protection. One of these added: 'I don't know what they do though. They can't stand outside all night waiting for the saucepan lids to be thrown'. Another said the police were a useful deterrent and another thought they could 'cool' the situation. One general practitioner advised contacting the Probation Office for legal help (in this case the Probation Service had an office within the health centre complex). One said the woman needed 'court backing', though he did not explain exactly what he meant by this. Another said he would take 'full notes for evidence'. Three thought that separation would be advisable, one of whom said: 'Leave him – inform the solicitor that *I've* advised this, then they're not deserting', a point made by one of the other doctors who advocated that the woman should leave her husband. Another thought the woman might want to leave but suggested 'an order' as an alternative. One specifically mentioned an injunction, saying, 'Suggest a lawyer and, if serious, get an injunction to keep the husband out'.

Despite this finding, as we pointed out in Chapter 6 we have other evidence to suggest that many general practitioners are cautious about becoming involved in their patients' domestic legal proceedings. Some view solicitors with a suspicion that occasionally verges on antagonism.

Discussion

It may be unrealistic to expect social workers, health visitors, and general practitioners to acquire a detailed knowledge of substantive law, since numerically marital violence is a marginal problem. But some practitioners do not even have an elementary understanding of legal matters. Consequently, some of their clients who are victims of marital violence and in need of legal help are plainly not getting it. It seems to us that some form of in-service training is required to make sure that these practitioners recognize the legal aspects of marital problems and know when to refer to a solicitor. This issue can be seen as symptomatic of a more fundamental problem of ignorance of relevant information. Here we are in the field of professional education and the need for a more inter-disciplinary approach so that the social evils of compartmental thinking can be avoided.

Notes

1 For a more critical appraisal of legal provision for victims of marital violence see Freeman 1979: 177–224.
2 For a fuller discussion of the role of police in marital violence, see T. Farragher, 'The Police and Marital Violence'; F. Wasoff, 'Violence to Women in the Home: a research strategy' – papers presented at DHSS Seminar on 'Violence in the Family – Recent Research on Services for Battered Women and their Children', University of Kent at Canterbury, September 1981; and L. Jeffery and J. Pahl, 'Battered Women and the Police' – paper given at the 1979 Conference of the British Sociological Association.
3 See, *Legal Action Group Bulletin:* 215, September, 1979.
4 For comment on the revised scheme see Freeman 1980.
5 S.1(2)(b) of the Act indicates that a person is defined as homeless if it is probable that occupation of accommodation 'will lead to violence from some other person residing in it or to threats of violence from some other person residing in it and likely to carry out the threat'. Subsequently a Code of Guidance was issued by the Department of the Environment, the Department of Health and Social Security, and the Welsh Office, asking housing authorities to 'respond sympathetically to applications from women who are in fear of violence'. During the passing of the Act it was argued that battered women should be one of the priority groups singled out by the Act as being in need of accommodation, as were pregnant women and one-parent families. However, this amendment was not passed.
6 It should be noted that the Housing Act 1980 has reduced the protection that local authorities can give battered wives. This Act, in the course of providing security of tenure for council tenants, has deprived councils of the power to take a violent male off the rent book and transfer the tenancy to the wife.
7 During our field-work, responsibility for homelessness was transferred from the Social Services Department, which in Bristol had a specialist section to deal with it, to the local Housing Authority.

10
Role definition

We set out to discover in general terms how practitioners saw their role when dealing with marital violence. In doing this we encountered a problem: practitioners found it extremely difficult to confine their remarks specifically to marital violence, partly because of the problem of defining the term marital violence, which we have already discussed, and partly because some practitioners did not have much experience of dealing with it. These considerations led us to adopt a broader focus and to consider the way practitioners viewed the scope and limitations of their role in dealing with *general* marital problems. In so doing, we were not able to check their definition against actual role performance in particular cases. We could not, therefore, expose any gaps between the ideal and the reality. Nevertheless, practitioners' statements may be indicative of the general yardstick they use when determining the extent of their responsibilities. We consider solicitors first.

Solicitors

INTRODUCTION

'As a professional group, solicitors probably have the most experience of marriages at the point of breakdown.' (Home Office Working Party on Marriage Guidance 1979)

The nub of a solicitor's formal role is to advise and, if need be, represent a client 'in the way that the solicitor thinks is best, using the utmost skill' on the client's behalf and 'acting with complete fairness towards him' (Council of the Law Society 1974). The adversary system of justice determines solicitors' partisan role, but some would argue that this general principle of partisanship requires qualification in practice, and needs to be modified where family matters are concerned (Mortlock 1971; Westcott 1977; Murch 1978). Solicitors and their clients sometimes argue that partisanship pursued unremittingly in family litigation may have adverse consequences, particularly for the relationships between children and parents. As the parties are likely to continue to be involved with each other after the legal issues of the case have been dealt with, the risk is that adversarial tactics will merely inflame already smouldering family relationships. O'Gorman (1963: 132–36) suggests that American lawyers recognize this, and mostly see themselves as counsellors seeking a fair settlement for both parties in matrimonial cases. Only a minority define their role in strictly partisan terms.

FINDINGS

In our feasibility study we discovered that if we asked solicitors merely to describe their role in matrimonial cases, virtually all gave a stock answer, namely to do their best for their client whether it be to advise or to represent in litigation.[1] In our main study we asked them more specific questions designed to probe deeper into the way they viewed their role. All were asked:

'In general, considering cases of marital violence, what kinds of help can you most effectively provide?'

The main point to emerge was that they saw themselves performing a wide range of tasks that involved a variety of roles, not only formally as the client's legal adviser and representative in court, but also informally, as the client's protector, confidant, counsellor, family friend, and occasionally, social worker. Sometimes they saw themselves as champions battling for their clients, sometimes as peacemakers restraining clients when their emotions boiled over and defied reason.

Individual solicitors differed in the emphasis they gave to these roles. Naturally, their response to the question was in part determined by the kind of clientele they worked with. Some lawyers, dealing with predominantly wealthy clients, have to spend much of their time sorting out financial and property matters that may be more serious and urgent if the wife is being assaulted. Others dealing with poorer clients find that they have to attend more to welfare problems and emergencies. Furthermore, the fact that they mentioned or emphasized particular features did not necessarily mean that other aspects would not have come into their definition had they had more time to reflect. For these reasons we decided that it would be mislead-

Role definition 137

ing to code and quantify their answers. It seemed better simply to illustrate the range of replies. They fall under the following headings.

Protector of legal rights

'You can only give practical legal help to ensure they suffer no further physical harm by using legal remedies such as injunctions, getting the husband out of the house etc. You obviously take proceedings, but you cannot ensure no further harm. An injunction is a piece of paper – it can help keep a bloke away but if he is determined to get her he will.'

The use of the law to obtain injunctions, divorce, etc. was of course the most usual initial reply to the question, despite frequently mentioned reservations about its effectiveness. Even so, there were many other aspects to their response. These are illustrated below.

Listener and 'diagnoser' of problems

There are two aspects to listening: it may be a help in itself; it may also be vital if the practitioner is to acquire the necessary information to advise properly:

'Sympathetic listening is a very large part of a legal practitioner's help – there may be no obvious legal remedies available to them that will work – you can only listen. They often don't realize that the law has its limitations. I put my watch on the table and listen for half-an-hour, then get on with the practical suggestions.'

Many solicitors pointed out that because victims of marital violence often come to them in agitated emotional states, it may take some time for the essence of the story to emerge, a point that can have financial policy implications for the Legal Advice Scheme:

'I'm very aware that as an employee of my firm I mustn't waste time. I find it is very difficult to give adequate time in these cases on the Green Form Scheme.[2] It almost forces one to cut out the sympathetic listening but I do stretch the limit to give them as much time as I can.'

Counsellor

Family lawyers these days stress the importance of what the Law Society has described as the solicitors' counselling role (Law Society

1977–78: 3). A number in our sample duly referred to it. Several remarked that they felt that in order to deal effectively with a client's legal problems they often first had to apply 'counselling' techniques to reduce the force of emotions clouding the client's perception of reality. For example, one remarked:

> 'The solicitor has two initial tasks – listening first and then counselling. It's very important to sort out the real fears from the illusory fears – the fact from the fantasy. You have to get her down from the high emotional level which she is often at when she comes in – that's important for the client and the lawyer. Then you can get on with the job of parting the two contestants – whether a firm letter of warning to the husband or an application to court for an injunction.'

Social worker

In 1968 Abel-Smith and Stevens suggested that in many respects the modern solicitor, like his Victorian counterpart a century ago, 'still acts as the social worker to the middle classes' (Abel-Smith and Stevens 1968: 146–47). These days with the Legal Aid and Advice Scheme, solicitors extend their particular brand of undercover social work to many working-class clients as well. Here are some illustrations of what might be termed practical social work activity:

> 'I look upon myself more as a social worker. Women are not worried about divorce, but about more pressing practical problems such as housing, money, sorting out the husband. That's more social work.'

> 'Giving legal advice is standard. Sometimes you have to do more than that – practical help. You may take them to the Women's Centre – I've done that twice. You can also do things like using the Green Form to get the locks changed – did you know that?'

> 'Practical help. I've occasionally jumped in the car with a battered wife and gone to her house to get clothes etc.'

Welfare rights advice

Almost all mentioned giving legal advice and explaining the legal remedies open to the client to deal with the violence. A number went further, and mentioned giving more general advice about welfare entitlements, an activity that solicitors are often criticized for not doing.

> 'Sorting out the welfare entitlements is a standard thing – supplementary benefit and all that. Social Services seem to have very limited resources and I've never found a voluntary agency that can help in those emergencies. It's no good just advising them to go to these places. I'm in the driving seat so I make appointments for them to go there.'

PARTISANSHIP OR NEUTRALITY?

All these informal tasks are performed from a standpoint of either traditional partisanship or neutrality. In order to identify what solicitors thought was their individual approach, we asked them the following question:

> 'Do you think a solicitor dealing with a marital dispute should take a neutral stance or be partisan?'

Table 10(1) quantifies their replies.

Table 10(1) *Solicitor's stance to marital dispute*

(n = 50)	%
Absolute partisanship	18
Qualified partisanship	26
Absolute neutrality	18
Qualified neutrality	24
A mixture of both – depending on circumstances	12
No reply	2

It will be noted that the sample was almost equally divided on the subject. They often felt strongly about the issue, suggesting considerable disagreement within the profession. Many of their replies criticized colleagues who took a contrary view on the matter. For example:

> 'I think your job is to get the most for your client and screw the other for what you can get.'

> 'You've got to be partisan. No man can listen to both sides and then do justice to their client.'

'I don't agree with being neutral – we are bred on the adversarial system – to do your client's bidding whether he be right or wrong, good or bad. Of course your non-violent matrimonial is now neutered to such an extent that one does in fact act neutrally. . . . But in a violent situation I get upset, though I shouldn't, and I get unpleasant. I have to pick up the pieces for this hopeless creature who doesn't know whether she is coming or going.'

This last comment betrays a not unusual degree of emotional identification with the client. Some argue that the professional discipline of legal education trains lawyers not to get emotionally involved. But nearly all the solicitors dealing with marital problems whom we interviewed acknowledged that the emotional pressures can be intense, sometimes affecting even the most experienced. Mortlock, himself a practising solicitor, has drawn attention to this point (1971: 162–70). Indeed, many of those suggesting a neutral stance argued that it helped them avoid emotional over-involvement. Here are some examples:

'You've got to be neutral for your own sanity. Nine times out of ten your client is giving as much as they are getting. You've got to look after your client's interests, but remain as objective as you can.'

'You can't give realistic, sound advice unless you can stand clear of the situation, so you've got to be neutral.'

'As I get more experienced I get more neutral. I used to get very involved.'

Apart from the minority who took an unqualified partisan stance, most acknowledged that their commitment to further their client's interests had to be balanced by other considerations, such as the interests of children in the family, the likely attitude of the court, and even the strength of the other side's case. All these interests can introduce conflicting obligations. Here are some examples:

'Where children are involved, you've got to set your client's interests on one side a little.'

'I see the problem in terms of the family, not just in the eyes of the spouse who comes to you. Things may seem very different through the eyes of a child.'

'You only get one side of the story from your client, but to do the job you must take the other side's case into account.'

Role definition 141

The conflicts faced by solicitors arise partly from the nature of the adversarial system of justice itself which 'sets the parties fighting' (Abraham 1962); and partly from the tendency of other solicitors to identify exclusively with their client's interests. The more a solicitor tries to be neutral, the more he is likely to be faced with conflicts of this kind, as can be seen in the following illustrations:

> 'It always annoys me when you get a case like this one [pointing to file on desk]. The other side's solicitor here has been absolutely intractable, refused to budge, absolutely no give and take. The result? He's driven a wedge between the parties needlessly and now we have a ridiculous squabble about every item of furniture.'

> 'Although people often want you to take their side initially, I think you should not. You should do all you can to bring down the emotional temperature because later you can give more realistic advice. But I can name three or four hard lawyers in this city who are hell to work with because their clients can never do any wrong.'

> 'I firmly believe that it is the job of the solicitor to work towards a situation which offers the best chance of happiness to all concerned. I don't like litigious lawyers. I find you particularly get this at the legal executive level. They haven't got the confidence to settle – they have to do everything by the book. They lack the self-confidence and discretion you find in most experienced qualified solicitors. It's hard to do business with them.'

SCOPE OF THE SOLICITOR'S ROLE

The question of partisanship or neutrality only partly exposes the way solicitors define the extent of their responsibility when dealing with clients' marital problems. In order to explore the matter further we asked them the following question:

> 'In cases of marital dispute does your responsibility lie only with the client or do you have added responsibility to other members of the family or to the court?'

Table 10(2) classifies their answers.

Virtually all solicitors said they had to consider the children, and to this extent children act as a constraint on the adoption of an extreme partisan position. But solicitors vary in how far they are prepared to go against their clients' wishes in order to safeguard the children's

Table 10(2) *Solicitor's view of responsibilities apart from client*

(n = 50)	%
Children and court	44
Children only	22
The whole family* and court	18
The family* only	10
Court only	6

* References to 'the family' include the other spouse as well as client and children.

interests. The following illustrations reveal some of the problems and show how practitioners try to reconcile the interests.

> 'My responsibility to the children particularly needs a lot of thought and care. I believe tugs of war over the children are extremely wrong. In those cases I sometimes have to give my client a verbal bashing over the head. In many cases that helps.'

> 'Children are a great problem. I suspect that I have more responsibility for the children than for the client in some cases. It produces a great conflict. I usually resolve it by saying to the client that I have a duty to tell the court all the facts.'

> 'The most difficult part of our job is getting clients to see sense about the children. They so often use them. Some clients would be horrified if they knew the limits solicitors go to in order to arrange something for the children.'

This practitioner was implying some behind-the-scenes 'fixing' with the other party's solicitor.

Even some of those solicitors who stressed that their primary responsibility was to their client said that if they thought the interest of client and child conflicted they might give up the case rather than try to accommodate both interests:

> 'My professional duty is first and foremost to my client. What I do is what they instruct me to do. If this is contrary to the interests of the children or the family I either do it or refuse to act.'

> 'It is impossible to do our job unless we stick to the principle that we are acting for the client. That responsibility is absolutely paramount. But I always put it to them that they must take into account

other members of the family such as the children. I try and guide them to be reasonable.'

The majority went further than this, adopting the view of the solicitor who told us:

> 'The client is very definitely *not* my only responsibility. I must consider the family as a whole, particularly the children. This is where family work differs from other litigation – even to the point of refusing to act for a client if I regard their instructions as damaging to the children.'

THE SOLICITOR'S DUTY TO THE COURT

Many mentioned their responsibility not to mislead the court knowingly, nor to waste its time. This is a basic principle of professional practice.[3] While some saw this as a rather academic point: 'I never forget that I'm an officer of the court, but I don't let it overburden me', others regarded it as a fundamental principle: 'You have an overriding duty not to mislead the court'; 'A solicitor's primary responsibility is to the court – no doubt about it. But you wouldn't believe that talking to some of our brethren and seeing how they perform!'.

Conflicting obligations to client and court may be more apparent than real. Clients may not always appreciate that their solicitor is furthering their interest by sticking by his duty to the court:

> 'I see my duty to present all the relevant evidence, even if it may seem a disadvantage to my client. Usually it will come out sooner or later – and it is always best to acknowledge it. This is where one's objectivity comes in. A solicitor also has to think of his credibility and reputation with the court.'

A number explained that their role as an officer of the court also helped them to protect the interests of children when these seemed at variance with their client's wishes: 'I will not put forward facts that I know to be false. One should acquaint the court with all the facts. Besides which, that also helps me discharge my duty to the children. I have to explain that to clients sometimes'.

SOLICITORS MEETING OTHER MEMBERS OF THE FAMILY

According to the evidence of divorcing parents, solicitors seldom see it as any part of their obligation to interview children and other members of the family (Murch 1978). One may assume this to be largely because of the risk of divided loyalty which threatens partisan commitment to the client. The Law Society's guide to professional practice states:

> 'Where a solicitor is concerned for two or more clients in non-contentious business, which might possibly become contentious, the solicitor must as soon as litigation is probable see that at least one of the clients is independently represented. If the solicitor would be embarrassed by reason of the knowledge that he had acquired of the case of the other client then he should see that both are separately advised.' (Council of the Law Society 1974)

During our feasibility study some solicitors said that they were prepared to interview children and, in certain circumstances, the other spouse. Thus, in the main study we asked:

> 'In marital disputes would you consider seeing (a) the other spouse and (b) the children?'

The other spouse

Table 10(3) quantifies the replies as they concern meeting the other spouse.

Table 10(3) *Whether solicitor would be prepared to meet other spouse*

(n = 50)	%
In no circumstances	28
Yes, initially together with my client	26
Yes, only if unrepresented	26
Yes, only if accompanied by solicitor	12
Yes – no reason given	8

Almost a third of the sample felt the risks of ethical problems arising from interviewing both parties were so great that they would never do it. They saw their role in strictly partisan terms:

> 'I won't allow it under any circumstances. You have got to have one-party interest. You can't view it both ways. I see my job as getting the best for my client. You can't do that if you take the other party into consideration.'

Role definition 145

'I would not see the other spouse. It is dangerous. You so easily get into a state of being a counsellor. It is not our function to arbitrate. Then if it breaks down you can't act for either because your own client loses confidence in you.'

'Even if they come in holding hands, you can't act for them. They *do* have conflicts of interests and the dangers are manifold if you try to act for both. You also run the risk of getting into an emotional tangle.'

Those who were prepared to see the other party gave various reasons. Sometimes they already knew both, for example through house purchase. In those circumstances they were usually prepared to give initial legal advice to couples contemplating separation:

'I'm willing to see both at an initial divorce meeting if they are both fairly intelligent people who want to do their best for the children. I explain to them their options and then send one or both off to see another solicitor.'

'I would see the other spouse where they both come in and say they want a divorce and it's all already agreed. I've also had meetings with the other spouse to try and get a reconciliation effected. But if it fails you may prejudice your position and have to send both to other solicitors.'

Some said they favoured 'round table' conferences where both parties, each accompanied by a legal representative, meet to negotiate settlement of various disputed matters. They were divided whether the practice was useful:

'Where the other spouse is represented I've found it helpful to try and arrange a meeting at a fairly early stage to talk things out. It's more difficult when the other spouse is not represented because they feel at a disadvantage and it is not a balanced discussion.'

'Occasionally I'll go to a round-table conference. I've never known it work to achieve a common objective, only ever seems to reinforce prejudices.'

Some occasionally seem to be willing to meet an unrepresented spouse but nearly always end up encouraging them to use another lawyer: 'I'll only see the other spouse if he is not represented and strictly on a party and party basis. "I act for your wife – I am not giving *you* advice". If they asked me for advice I would probably tell them to get their own solicitor first'.

Sometimes their client wants them to meet the other spouse. In those circumstances some solicitors agree:

> 'I would say, "I'm acting for your wife. I'm seeing you because she wants it and you do. I can't advise you. You must get separate advice". The cases I'm thinking of are nearly always repentant violent husbands who plead with the lawyer to persuade her back.'

Seeing the children

Table 10(4) quantifies the solicitors' replies to the question whether they would consider seeing children when dealing with marital cases.

Table 10(4) *Whether solicitor would be prepared to see children*

(n = 50)	%
Yes	34
Yes – qualified. Older ones only	22
Yes – but only casually if accompanying a parent	12
No	32

A few who said they would, argued that it helped them get an overall view of the case, and to appreciate the children's position better:

> 'I often see the children – their interests are paramount. It can give you considerable insight. You have to be open-minded and never assume your client can do no wrong.'

> 'If I'm acting for the parent seeking custody I always see the children at some point.'

The majority of solicitors were cautious about seeing the children:

> 'I am reluctant to do it. I don't have that much experience with children and wouldn't be too happy about being able to interpret what they say.'

> 'I might see children – say from about eight years onwards. The problem is children always try to say what they think you want them to say – so I'm not sure you get at the truth.'

Role definition 147

'Mothers often bring the smaller ones. I don't like the older ones hearing all the gory details. The presence of a child can often constrain a mother from telling you what you need to know.'

'I will see them on occasions, but I don't like bringing the kids into it. Could be trouble with professional etiquette. The other solicitor might be aggrieved that I had seen them.'

Solicitors disagreed about calling children as witnesses in cases of marital violence.

'I try and avoid seeing the children. It's likely to have a bad effect on them involving them further in the matrimonial dispute. Even if they are subject to dispute I don't want to be seen as influencing them in any way. I'd also be extremely reluctant to use them as witnesses to marital violence.'

'Generally, the less children are involved the better. I would never call them in to take sides. Might see a teenager if they want to say who they wish to live with. Sometimes, if they have been victims of violence as well I need to see them.'

Local authority social workers

INTRODUCTION

Social Service Departments do not specialize in the treatment of marital problems, although some of their staff may have studied the sociology of marriage and the nature of marital interaction quite deeply.[4] Mattinson and Sinclair (1979) confirm our own findings (in Chapter 2) that the proportion of cases presenting overt marital problems to Social Service Departments is comparatively small although often acute.[5] Social workers often become aware of clients' marital problems in the context of their other work – for example dealing with juvenile delinquency, child neglect, homelessness, mental illness, the care of the handicapped and aged. Some social workers are 'caseworkers' trained to work in depth with the emotionally interactive components of marital and family relationships. Others, probably the majority, see their role in broader, less intensive terms, often focusing more on the clients' material needs. The way they define their role is partly conditioned by the priorities of departmental policy, and partly by their experience, the kind of training they have received, and their personal inclination. These elements sometimes harmonize and reinforce the role adopted; at other times they contradict one another. Practitioners' management of these elements will be partly determined by the scope of the discretion they feel they have.

FINDINGS

We did not ask social workers to describe their role in marital cases. Our experience during our feasibility study suggested that the social workers' answers would be too diverse and insufficiently exclusive of one another to quantify. We decided it would be better to explore their conception of role by asking:

> 'A couple come to Social Services asking for help with marital difficulties – minimal violence but serious relationship problems. How would they be dealt with?'

Table 10(5) indicates the general nature of the replies.

Table 10(5) *Couple approaching agency with marital problem*

(n = 50)	%
Would take it on initially anyway	38
Would take it on, only if children involved	20
Would refer to Marriage Guidance	38
No reply	4

Nearly all remarked that it would be rare for a couple to approach the department with such a request. Even if they did, there would be only a small chance of meeting a social worker sufficiently interested and with the time to offer marital or family therapy. An exception might be where there were children who were clearly at risk.

Those confident in their casework skills said they might take the case on, but they usually qualified their reply:

> 'I would take them on for counselling whether or not they had children, but only if I wasn't overloaded with statutory duties.'

> 'I personally would like to offer the couple a contract[6] over a defined period of time, say six sessions. Some of my colleagues would immediately think of Marriage Guidance, especially if they were up to their necks in child-care cases. We tend to get shot of things to other agencies if we can.'

Nineteen said they would refer the case to Marriage Guidance, some reluctantly, others justifying it on the grounds that Marriage Guidance Counsellors had more appropriate skills to offer, or more time. A number pointed out that a great deal would depend on the inclination of the social workers and the state of staff resources in their particular team.

'It would depend on who saw them. Social workers have different interests. When I first came to this area this kind of case would go by the board – too busy for it, so suggest MG. Now some of us might be inclined to take them on. We have become a little more specialist and we have one or two social workers who are into marriage guidance and family therapy.'

Neutrality or partisanship?

All social workers were asked:

'In a marital dispute do you feel you should take a neutral stance or be partisan?'

The great majority said that in theory they *should* be neutral but that in practice they were partisan to the woman because they tended to have more contact with her and usually saw her as the weaker partner.

In order to examine how they saw themselves in relation to male partners, we asked:

'In cases of marital dispute do you ever see the men?'

Twenty-nine reported usually doing so. Of the remainder, eight said that the husbands were normally not willing to talk about their problems, and four remarked that the wives were usually reluctant for them to meet the husband. The age or sex of the social worker and the timing of the visit were all advanced as important factors determining whether the husband was seen. For example a forty-year-old male social worker remarked: 'I see the men in a lot of these cases. Being a male social worker, it's easier for men to identify with me and to believe that I will accept their point of view more readily. I'm afraid this seems particularly true of those men who see wives as second-rate citizens'.

A younger woman social worker made the same point in a different way: 'Often the men are at home when I call in the evenings but they seem reluctant to see me. Maybe it's because I'm young (twenty-three) and female that they find it hard to accept my role as social worker. I have to make a real effort to get them involved'. A young male social worker remarked:

> 'I find it's a bit of a problem with the men – my age comes into it if they are older than I am. Men are so much more elusive. Apart from anything else, we work nine to five most of the time. We see the wives more often and the men tend therefore to see us as the wives' social worker and not as the family social worker.'

Several observed that women talked more easily about marital problems than men:

> 'I work more closely with women because women express their problems more readily than men. I wouldn't want to collude with them and point the finger at men, but it just seems that often the men don't want to talk anyway. Either it's an infringement of his privacy, a slight to his self-respect, or he just isn't used to talking about problems like this.'

Children

All social workers were asked:

'In cases of marital dispute do you ever see the children?'

Table 10(6) classifies the replies.

Table 10(6) *Whether social workers would see children*

(n = 50)	%
Yes	24
Yes, if older	26
Yes, if they're around	4
Yes, in the later stages	12
No	28
No response	6

Two-thirds favoured seeing children, especially if they were old enough:

> 'I prefer to talk with the children as well as parents as a way of opening up family communications about things like that. I think it's beneficial. A child can be very tormented when parents, who are often the sole providers of its welfare, are at loggerheads. Talking with the children about it can help them express their anxieties and

help them feel that someone else cares and has another perspective to offer them.'

Many who took this view were inclined to redefine the couple's marital problem as a wider family one, several pointing out that some parents tried to conceal their problems from the children: 'Generally speaking it's the more educated responsible parents who don't want the children to know. These wives often seem to be protecting their husband's image – don't want the children to know what their father is like'. A few social workers saw themselves as family therapists:

'I do some family therapy. It's helpful to open up these concealed marital difficulties so that all the family can see that nothing terrible happens if you do talk about things in the open. Often this relieves the tension in the children. Sometimes I've found that older children can provide a perspective which up to then the parents have not been able to see.'

Another remarked: 'Discussion with all the family members of problems that exist, but are not usually recognized, is valuable. It helps to get at the things which might lie behind the children's difficulties'. Some saw family therapy as a particularly appropriate way of dealing with marital violence: 'The majority of violent marriages are a family thing and it's therefore appropriate to work with the family as a whole. I think it is useful for the parents to know what the children know and feel'.

The minority of social workers who did not favour talking with children advanced similar reasons to those given by solicitors:

'I wouldn't do so deliberately unless a teenager brought it up. If they have witnessed violence it's probably traumatic enough without being asked to relive it.'

'Parents generally don't want you speaking to their children. Unless they are old enough they would feel threatened speaking to strangers about something that might terrify them. It's also so easy to influence children against their parents.'

Health Visitors

INTRODUCTION

The delivery of domiciliary public health care is normally[7] divided in the United Kingdom between district nursing sisters, who provide basic nursing care, and health visitors, 'who deal exclusively in prevention, giving advice on health and social problems, and in case-finding for more specialized agencies such as those involved in intensive social case-work' (Dingwall 1971: 21). All health visitors are registered nurses with obstetric experience, and hold the Health Visitors' Certificate. They have a statutory duty to visit routinely all mothers with children under five, to advise on child-rearing problems, although they have no right of entry. They have discretion to decide how often to visit. Unlike social workers, they have a major commitment to visit normal, healthy, coping families. They generally feel that they should not neglect this duty by getting drawn into intensive social work with the problem minority.

In Bristol, as elsewhere, they have taken on the task of visiting the elderly, advising them on medical and social problems. They have also developed a specific liaison role with general medical practitioners. Attachments to groups of doctors now form the basis of their organization, having replaced the older system based on geographical area.

Health visitors and general practitioners are intended to form part of a primary health care team, each having equal status 'with distinct and complementary spheres of competence' (Dingwall 1971: 214). At the time of our research it was clear that in some instances the aims of this scheme were not being achieved. Some GPs do not regard health visitors as equals, seeing them as ancillary medical aides working under their direction. There is some conflict here about how each occupation defines the role of the other, unless health visitors themselves agree they are not the doctors' equals. This issue is discussed more fully in the next chapter. We mention it here because it sometimes influenced the way health visitors answered the question:

> 'How do you see your role in relation to your patients' marital problems?'

FINDINGS

It should be borne in mind that unlike the other three occupations in our study, health visitors nearly always take the initiative to contact their clients, at least until they have established a relationship with them. In contrast to the other groups, they were fairly well agreed about their role when dealing with marital problems: basically to be a sympathetic listener – primarily to the wife – and source of supportive advice and practical help for her. The majority (thirty-one) saw their role as largely confined to listening. Most of the others, usually the more experienced and confident, saw it in more active terms, for example giving advice and information about social welfare provisions; sometimes offering practical help of various kinds as well as arranging referral to more specialist agencies. A few said they would offer short-term counselling. Health visitors drew a distinction between listening, which they did so much of themselves, and counselling which they saw as an activity more usually performed by social workers and Marriage Guidance counsellors. It may well be that the modest person's 'listening' is the pretentious person's 'counselling'.

The modest way in which health visitors define their role may reflect a relatively low evaluation which they ascribe to their functions in comparison with the way they see GPs. Other research (Dingwall 1971) has commented on this, seeing it as a feature of nurses' traditional deference to doctors. It may mask considerable self-confidence.

Supportive listening

Most took a positive view of their role as sympathetic listeners:

> 'Sympathetic listening is the main thing because often there's no-one in their family or friends they can talk to. They can't talk to mother, wouldn't want her to know, and friends would talk about it. It's mainly the wives because I don't see the husbands much. I'm always amazed how often they say, "Just talking to you seems to help". The trouble is you come back weighed down with it and feel mentally exhausted.'

> 'Being a good listener is the main part of our work, but I suppose it's more than that really because it's guiding them to see what their problem really is. It's sitting down with them and clarifying the options that they can follow for themselves.'

Health visitors themselves stress that the primary value of listening is that it may have a directly cathartic value to mothers. But it must not be forgotten that much of the health visitor's work consists of quietly and benignly carrying out family surveillance aimed at safeguarding the interests of children. Much of their skill lies in gathering information about the family which is 'converted into records or stored in their heads' (Dingwall 1971: 86). It may be used later for reports to other services or other members of the primary health care team.

Social welfare

As we have seen, health visitors, rather more than doctors and solicitors, tend to explain marital problems and violence as reactions to environmentally induced stress – poor housing conditions, poverty, unemployment, and physical illness. To some extent this tends to be reflected in the way they define their role in relation to such problems. A number emphasized the practical things they wanted to do.

> 'I can find money or food at a pinch, get clothes and spare furniture from WRVS, arrange help from the churches like interest-free loans. I can take pressure off the mother by getting the toddler into a day nursery or even set the wheels in motion for a child to go into care. Practical help can mean so much more to someone really stressed than a lot of sympathetic talk.'

> 'I often feel I'd like to go in and roll up my sleeves and tidy things up, but you have to be careful who you do that for. They can sit and wait for you to come and do the same again next time.'

Some of those who mentioned providing practical help seemed almost apologetic about it, as if they regarded it as an 'unprofessional' activity. Confirmation of this came from several of the more senior health visitors. For example, one said:

> 'I think we should be supportive without being benevolent. So many young health visitors think you should find money, gifts of food etc. That is not the answer to marital problems. It's the easy way out to say to a mother, "You need £15 for a holiday". What they need is *time* to talk to someone. Time is the big thing. It's so important to let them feel you are not hurried, even if you are.'

Liaison with other services

Health visitors see liaising between families and other services as a major part of their role. We were told repeatedly that linking up people with the resources available, mainly from other health and social services, was part of their general 'supportive' role. They try to work closely with their local general practitioners and social workers.

The provision of long-term support is one of the ways in which health visitors differentiate their role from local authority social workers. Continuity of long-term care to families places them in a good position to expedite the delivery of more specialist services:

'Often we are very much the centre link between other agencies simply because we are the one continuing agency. We go on visiting for a long time after the crisis situation, which the social worker may have dealt with, has blown over. This continuing support is the strength of our work.'

Health visitors stress that their long-term preventive work is with the 'general' population, whereas they see social workers as dealing with the crises of people with serious social problems: 'We see everybody – the normal plus the "problem families". We can therefore get a more balanced view of things'. They try to prevent the deterioration which would otherwise throw up problems for social workers later.

Marital counselling

Some experienced health visitors said they did counselling in the client's home which they saw as an advantage over other services:

'So often the young couples don't talk to one another about the emotional side of things. Talking to us enables the mothers to vocalize their thoughts and feelings. Given time you can often help them appreciate their partner's point of view better.'

They also argued that people fought shy of going to a special place for counselling. Yet most health visitors did not seem particularly confident about counselling, usually suggesting that more specialist services would have greater skills to offer if only the mother or the couple would go to them. 'As far as one is able to, one should do counselling, but one must know one's limitations. If one is out of one's depth you have to refer to other agencies.'

The scope of health visitors' responsibility in cases of marital violence

All health visitors were asked:

'In cases of marital violence – apart from the child – whose interests do you consider most?'

The majority (37/50) thought that apart from children, the mother was their main concern. The reasons advanced were rather what one would expect from a service primarily concerned with mothers of infant children.

'The mother, because I see her more than the husband. The family as a whole is important, but I see it through the eyes of the wife.'

'Instinctively the person being battered – nearly always the mother. She's the one I'm most involved with and they seem more vulnerable than the men. She doesn't hold the power/money, so she's usually the weaker of the two.'

'The mother. She's the head of the family in most cases – she takes on most responsibility, so our duty is to support and protect her.'

The remainder mainly said that they tried to be neutral. Even so, most of these acknowledged the pressures to take up a partisan role in favour of the mother. Thus one remarked:

'I'd like to be neutral but it's usually the wife I'm concerned about most, simply because she is the one I meet most. I know that's biased, one-sided, and not very fair, since the husbands usually need as much help as she does in the long term to get their aggression more under control.'

Overall, most implied that their partisan commitment to the mother placed severe limitations on any attempt to help the couple together. One told us that it could be frightening encountering a husband who saw her as being on the wife's side.

'I had one chasing me round a housing estate because he thought I told his wife to leave. Husbands get aggressive because they know the wife has talked to you, think you are on her side. They feel insulted as if it's a slight on their manliness, a sign of weakness or something to have a marital problem.'

The health visitor who made the following remark was exceptional in her capacity to see herself in a neutral role:

'The interest of the child is the main criterion. You need a happy family to make a happy child, therefore you've got to consider both mother *and* father. One can't take mother's side all the time. It's often six of one and half-a-dozen of the other when you really look into it.'

Possibly more would agree with the health visitor who said: 'The children come first, the mother second. Children need a mother, however bad she is. Most families can get by without a dad'. While this view may well be realistic, it is perhaps worth noting that when asked whether they had ever talked with the husbands in cases where they knew of marital problems, only a minority (thirteen) said that they would make a standard practice of trying to do so. Of the remaining thirty-seven, twenty said that they would do so if they met the husband by chance, and that this happened only occasionally; seventeen said that they hardly ever met the husbands in those circumstances and would certainly not attempt to do so.

Various points emerged from their answers to this question. Some clearly saw the GP as more appropriate to talk to the husband sometimes on the basis that a 'man prefers to talk to a man', sometimes because they thought that the man would feel they were already biased in favour of the wife. Several mentioned that wives could be reluctant for them to talk with the husband. One said:

'I always ask the wife if she would agree to my having a word with her husband or seeing them together, but the wives are usually against it: "No, no, he wouldn't want to talk to you". I think the wives more often tell you of their problems just to let you know – they don't want you to do anything about it.'

Another said: 'I usually ask but they say it's no use. I suggest MGC and they say, "He'd never go" '.

In assessing these last two comments, it should be remembered that the health visitor is in a different position from the other three occupations because of her routine visiting. You do not have to go to her with a defined problem. She comes along, and if you are feeling miserable and she has the time, you can talk to her even if you do not want anything done.

A few health visitors who claimed to be successful in meeting husbands apparently have a policy about it. They try to meet young fathers as soon as they can after the baby is born. In this way they build up a relationship with both parents. Nevertheless, most acknowledged that unless the husbands are unemployed and at home when they visit during the day, they usually have little chance to speak to them. A few said that they would make a special evening visit to see a couple together or to talk with a father on his own, but on the whole more thought this would involve a degree of intensive work best left to a social worker or someone else.

General medical practitioners

INTRODUCTION

Doctors disagree about whether they should define their role narrowly or broadly when dealing with their patients' marital problems. Some feel that they should limit themselves to strictly medical aspects. Others think that they should concern themselves with related social and psychological matters as well. We will illustrate various aspects of this disagreement and offer some explanations for it. We should point out that patients, and also other interested professionals such as social workers and health visitors, generally agree with doctors who take the broad view.

In our representative study of divorcing parents conducted in Bristol in 1972, it was found that 55 per cent of the women and 42 per cent of the men had been to see their GP about their marriage problems, whereas the respective figures for the next most popular service, the local authority social services, were 13 per cent and 10 per cent. As will be seen in *Table 10(7)*, it was also found that, apart from solicitors,[8] general practitioners were seen as the most helpful of all services, either statutory or voluntary.[9]

Table 10(7) *Social caretakers found most helpful (Bristol Divorce Research 1972–75)*

	Divorce petitioners (n = 102)		
	Men (n = 31) %	Women (n = 71) %	Total %
No-one consulted	36	27	30
Doctor	29	42	38
Local Authority Social Worker	3	6	5
Probation Officer	–	3	2
Minister of Religion	3	1	2
Marriage Guidance Counsellor	–	2	1
Others (school-teacher, voluntary social worker, etc.)	3	6	5
None reported helpful	26	13	17

Divorcing parents gave a number of reasons why they went to the doctor about their marital problems and why they mostly found it helpful. Many had sought treatment for physical and psychiatric symptoms which they attributed to the stress of their marriage break-up.[10] Many also reported that they had sought the doctor's general advice about how they should deal with their marital problems. They saw the doctor as able to provide sympathetic advice in a confidential, non-stigmatic way. The majority were pleased with the help received, some remarking that the doctor had made special appointments for them at the end of surgery hours so as to allow them more time.

The Dobashes' Scottish study of 109 women who had been to refuges showed that doctors were more likely to be approached than any other service (Dobash and Dobash 1980: 249). Pahl's English study of fifty women interviewed at a refuge for battered women found that thirty-two had consulted their doctor about their marital problems and about the violent behaviour of the man with whom they were living. Of these the majority (56 per cent) had said that the doctor had been helpful. These women liked best the doctors who: 'listened carefully, approached the problem sympathetically, offered appropriate advice, both medical and non-medical'. The most frequently reported medical response found 'unhelpful' was the 'prescribing of anti-depressants and tranquillizers, most commonly valium'. Pahl writes that many women saw such 'treatment as an inappropriate stop-gap measure which could well postpone their achievement of a satisfactory long-term solution' of their problems (Pahl 1979).

Of course, women who have defined themselves as 'battered' and have sought refuge may not be comparable with a cross-section of women divorce petitioners or even of other victims of marital violence who stay in their marriages, and who may not seek any help. Nevertheless, such consumer evidence as exists from selective samples such as these, emphasizes the importance of a sympathetic doctor. We agree, therefore, with the following assertion made by the Home Office Working Party on Marriage Guidance:

> 'the family doctor is seen by most people as the all-purpose person to turn to in any difficulties which are remotely connected with pain or ill health; this depends not only upon the personalities of doctor and patient but also upon cultural factors. Marital tensions produce stress symptoms in so many couples that it is scarcely surprising that the family doctor is frequently consulted . . . about the whole range of emotional, sexual and relationship difficulties.' (Home Office Working Party on Marriage Guidance 1979: 43)

While we know that the total number of consultations of this kind must be fairly high, it has not been quantified. This is because the standard tools of epidemiology, as the Royal College of General Practitioners has pointed out, do not provide an adequate classification system. The result is that 'the presentation of marital problems is hidden in medical statistics under a variety of morbidity labels. . . . Marital unhappiness can present as depression, as a headache or backache, or a heavy period or a child who refuses to go to school' (Home Office Working Party on Marriage Guidance 1979: 145). It seems clear that practitioners who define their role narrowly may well be at variance with many of their patients who expect them to define it broadly.

FINDINGS

Each general practitioner in our survey was asked:
 'How do you see your role when patients tell you of their marital problems?'
Not surprisingly, all said that they would deal with medical problems such as cuts, bruises, and other injuries arising from marital violence; psycho-sexual problems, and psychiatric states, such as depression or anxiety arising from stress. We then probed to see whether the doctors would define their role more broadly, for example in terms of offering advice and counselling. Approximately half were willing to do so, while the others said they restricted themselves to medical rather than psycho-social help.

In general it seemed as if doctors' perception of role depended a great deal on the way they understood the nature of marital problems. They appeared most at ease when they could justify their activities in terms of treating illness. In our opinion, the doctors' definition of what constitutes illness is crucial to the way they define their role. In general, provided they can see marital problems in medically dysfunctional or pathological terms, they are quite happy about having a go at dealing with them. But if they cannot, they nearly always express doubts about their role. If they see marital problems primarily in social or economic rather than mental health terms, they are likely to define their role narrowly and say that other services, such as those provided by social workers or health visitors, are better suited to deal with them. Some doctors felt that although marital problems are basically social rather than medical in character, they could often do a better job than the social services, who were seen as under-staffed and over-worked.

Various reasons were advanced by those who defined their role broadly. There were those who said that doctors often had established relationships with patients, were often trusted with confidences, and were thus in a strong position to offer general advice:

'I do a lot of ante-natal counselling especially with the first child, because I think that is one of the points when you can prevent marital disharmony. I concentrate on the women, offer them common-sense advice to help them appreciate the father's role. Anyone can do the kinds of things I do, but I have the entry as a doctor and the weight.'

Some doctors, usually those who had practised a number of years in the same area, saw themselves as family friends, almost father confessors:

'I cherish the concept of family doctor rather than general practitioner. In positive terms I enjoy involvement with the family as a whole. The doctor has a natural supportive link with the family, is trusted, and is privy to many family secrets. He can look into the family situation. It's important to take this role on, and not pass it on to some ancillary medical worker who would probably be over-worked anyway.'

'I hope my patients see me as counsellor and friend. I suppose I have what is looked upon these days as an old-fashioned practice. My patients don't find me writing their prescriptions as they walk in. I want my patients to come to me with a problem if they wish, and to feel able to talk openly about it.'

One or two were not averse to playing the role of family policeman:

'If there is violence you have to be a bit of a policeman and keep an eye on it. You have to be prepared to intervene sometimes without permission.'

'The police are usually reluctant to interfere. They call for me. I don't take sides and don't interfere unnecessarily. By the time I see the husband he's contrite, but I say what I think – that it's mean, cowardly, and horrid to hit a woman.'

A number said that they saw themselves as marriage counsellors:

'We get a lot of these problems. I used to send people hopefully to the MGC but it's miles away and both partners usually won't go. Anyhow, patients usually translate their marital problem into medical terms. I see my job these days as to translate it back.'

'I try to see where the root of their problems lie. Helping them define their problem is what I'm here for. I would say in about 40 per cent of the cases coming in with physical symptoms I become aware of underlying problems. Like a marriage guidance counsellor, I ask myself, "Are they putting the blame on their partner?" when that isn't the root of their problem.'

Some thought that they had other advantages over Marriage Guidance: 'Patients see the doctor as having more authority and more weight than a marriage guidance counsellor, I think the doctor has a positive role in helping with sexual problems, loss of libido during the menopause, etc.'.

These comments imply that some patients find it easier to present marital problems covertly as medical problems. They also imply that some patients would rather talk to their trusted doctor than to an unfamiliar marriage guidance counsellor or social worker. Of course, they may well feel subconsciously that they can only be sure of getting the doctor's ear if they can present some physical symptoms. A sizeable minority of doctors, recognizing this, seemed willing to take on a counselling role designed to help patients decide their marital future with greater understanding: 'I see my role as a counsellor who lets them talk out their problems and help *them* make decisions. I don't make decisions for them'.

Doctors who took a broad view of their role, acknowledged that sympathetic listening could of itself be a therapeutic way of relieving a patient's anxieties:

'It helps to be a good listener. When I was young, I was appalled by confidences. Having worried for a week, when they came in next time I'd ask timidly how things were and then they'd say, "It's all right. You helped by listening". You hadn't done much but having told someone they felt better able to cope.'

Yet for every doctor who suggested this point of view, there was another who thought that the relatively passive role of being a sympathetic listener was inappropriate. Many of these saw their role in strictly medical treatment terms. They were inclined to argue that work-loads allowed them insufficient time to go into the details of patients' marital problems or to attempt counselling. Even where they saw a need for such approaches they generally remarked that it was better for somebody else with more time available to do it: 'It needs a tremendous amount of talking to partners concerned – it's much too time-consuming. My health visitor can be more help than I. She has the time to discuss'.

Role definition 163

A few also pointed out that they were not trained to deal with the wider aspect of marital problems:

'I feel very inadequate when faced with so many of these behaviour problems. I have a lot of difficulty dealing with two partners. I confess it's easier to take the side of one and agree that the other is in the wrong. I really cannot deal with this sort of thing – not trained to do it. Perhaps medical students are better trained now than in my day.'

The scope of the doctor's responsibility

Like solicitors and practitioners in other services, doctors define their role in dealing with their patients' marital problems not only in terms of the range of response they might make, but also in terms of the people they include within the scope of their responsibility. In order to explore this, we asked:

'In cases of marital dispute does your responsibility lie only with the patient or do you have added responsibility to other members of the family?'

Only four said unequivocally that they would limit their responsibility to the individual patient presenting the problem. Most of the remainder said that they had responsibility to children of the family and sometimes to the other marital partner, especially if on their medical list.

In order to see whether these doctors would be prepared to translate their concern for other members of the family into action, we asked them whether they would normally consider seeing the children or other spouse in marital disputes. *Table 10(8)* summarizes their replies.

Table 10(8) *Whether doctor would normally consider seeing: (a) children of the family; (b) other partner, in marital disputes (n = 50)*

(a) Children	%	(b) Other partner	%
Would *not* see children	34	Would *not* see other partner	12
Would occasionally see children	36	Would see other partner	56
Would normally see children	22	Ideally would try to see other partner but they usually refuse	26
Would ask health visitor to see children	4		
No reply	4	No reply	6

Children

Most of those who said that they would consider seeing children qualified their reply by saying that they would only normally see teenagers:

> 'Wouldn't see them when they were very young. If there was a great deal of violence going on I might visit them to see if they were OK.'

> 'It depends on their age entirely. Children under five or seven will not be aware of what goes on. With a teenager – say thirteen to fifteen – it could make a considerable difference. That's the age when kids go off the rails, particularly if there is no support behind them. The younger ones might come to surgery with enuresis problems. I always have to consider what's going on at home.'

The need to avoid upsetting children further was the most commonly advanced reason for not seeing them: 'I don't discuss it with the children, no. They've been traumatized enough. It would be different if they wanted to see me, but I can't think of a case'. Our overall impression was that doctors seldom make a point of seeing children.

The other partner

The majority said that they would consider taking the initiative to see the other partner. Whether in fact they normally do so is hard to say. Nevertheless, their replies are important, since they suggest that doctors see their role in terms of the couple rather than the individual patient when dealing with marital problems. Even so, many indicated that it was relatively unusual for the other partner, by inference usually the man, to be willing to be seen. 'They very rarely turn up – they feel they are going to be told off.' One commented that as it was usually the wife who had seen the doctor first, the husband could easily feel that the doctor had become prejudiced in her favour. Another pointed out that he could only ask to see the other partner provided he was on his medical list: 'You have to be careful here. It raises an important point of medical ethics. You should never divulge information given to you by one partner to the other without permission. Therefore you can only see the husband if the wife has given permission'.

Some preferred seeing both partners together to get a more balanced view of things and to avoid some of these ethical difficulties:

'I normally try to make joint appointments. I don't believe in hearing one-sided stories. You need to see both together if you are going to be a mediator'. Whether husbands were seen could depend on how firm the doctor was in making the approach. One or two were surprisingly robust, particularly if marital violence was involved: 'I always ask to see them and in my experience they usually come. They seldom tell you straight what's been going on – but they know you know. If they won't come in, then I go to them – visit or 'phone. In bad cases I warn them that if necessary I'll go to the police'.

We discuss the policy significance of the respective roles of solicitors, local authority social workers, health visitors, and general medical practitioners in Chapter 12.

Notes

1 There were of course minor variations, but this was the main gist of the answers.
2 Legal Aid Act 1974, see 2(1). The Legal Advice Scheme allows a solicitor to give advice and assistance 'in the application of English Law to any particular circumstances which have arisen in relation to the person seeking the advice'. The solicitor completes a green application form to claim reimbursement from the Legal Aid fund – hence the term 'Green Form Scheme'.
3 See Council of the Law Society (1974). The practitioners' guide points out that:
'this can involve the advocate in difficult questions of professional responsibility. The proper administration of justice requires that the court should be able to rely on lawyers who appear before it or have dealings with it. There must be no deception of the court in relation to anything which the court is required to know. . . . A solicitor must no keep back from the court any information within his knowledge which the court is entitled to have before it.'
4 See Home Office Working Party on Marriage Guidance (1979). This report states:
'The Association of Directors of Social Services thought that Social Service Departments ought in future to equip themselves to the role to help with problems revealed in a situation with which they were already dealing, but they could not in the foreseeable future provide a service for marital counselling as such.'
5 See Mattinson and Sinclair (1979). The authors write:
'From the study of 1198 cases two things are clear. Firstly at the intake stage the number of cases having an overt marital problem was very small. In only 3% of the total did the social workers think it worth while

mentioning a marital problem on the referral sheet. Secondly with negligible exceptions those who had overt marital problems neither referred themselves nor were referred with an overt request to deal with the marital problem for its own sake. Battered wives required accommodation and deserted husbands day care facilities for children . . . but this was a far cry from requesting the social worker to intervene in their marital affairs.'

6 Social worker here was probably referring to a particular method of time-focused social casework. See Reid and Shyne 1969.
7 In some areas there are joint appointments.
8 See Murch (1978), 'The Role of Solicitors in Divorce Proceedings'. Sixty per cent of this sample of divorcing parents reported that they were either satisfied or very satisfied with their solicitor. At the time this survey was made virtually all divorce petitioners consulted lawyers.
9 Similar findings for the divorcing population are reported by Mitchell (1981) and Chester (1973).
10 Depression was the most common symptom (63 per cent of women and 45 per cent of men). Other symptoms included sleeplessness (10 per cent men, 4 per cent women), weight loss (7 per cent men, 11 per cent women), skin troubles (3 per cent men, 1 per cent women), stomach upsets, ulcers etc. (3 per cent men, 0 per cent women).

11
Perceptions of other services

Introduction

When exploring the needs of clients from violent partnerships, practitioners should consider whether referral to another service is appropriate. Their decision will be influenced by their knowledge of other services and their confidence in them. In this Chapter we explore this issue by examining the way the four practitioner groups viewed each other's role as well as the role of Marriage Guidance and Women's Aid, specialist services designed to deal with different aspects of marital problems.

In reporting practitioners' views of other services several things must be remembered: their opinions may be based on myth or hearsay rather than on direct experience. Moreover, as Miller has pointed out: 'Frequently individuals in one agency are unclear as to the role and competence of other agencies which might be seen as responsible for handling a particular aspect of the problem' (Miller 1975: 28). Mattinson and Sinclair suggest that there may be something in the nature of work with marital conflict that sets one practitioner or service against another. The dynamic of conflict invites outsiders to take sides. Troubled people may have idealized expectations of the help that should be available to them. Similarly, practitioners may have idealized expectations of other services (Mattinson and Sinclair 1979: 275, 283).

One should also bear in mind that partnerships that deteriorate to the point of breakdown may have a long career of violence during the course of which the parties' needs may change. The Dobashes have suggested that initially, battered wives are likely to want their marriage to continue. Later, as things get worse, they want external authority to challenge the man's use of violence. Finally, they seek escape and help in ending the relationship (Dobash, Dobash, and Cavanagh 1981). Very often GPs are the first service to be approached. Solicitors tend to come in to the picture only in the later stages of marriage breakdown or when the violence has become intolerable. Practitioners may not appreciate the significance of the client's choice of service, including their own. We examine the changing pattern of help-seeking further in Chapter 12.

Profound problems arise from differences of professional ethos. Doctors committed to preserving marriage and to thinking in terms of cure, may look askance at solicitors whom they may see as speeding people to divorce. Some practitioners feel suspicious, indeed antagonized by what they see as the militant feminism of women who run refuges. There are other ways in which differences of professional ethos can affect collaboration between services. For example, those who place a high premium on confidentiality, such as solicitors and doctors, may be cautious about working with services that take a more pragmatic view. Also, practitioners, like many clients, might resist close association with services considered stigmatic.

All these matters affect the state of diplomatic relationships within the complex web of services involved with marital partnerships. We have not been able to explore them comprehensively. However, we became convinced that powerful, if somewhat hidden, forces influence the way practitioners discriminate between services. These can be too easily ignored by those who glibly indulge in collaboration rhetoric (Home Office Working Party on Marriage Guidance 1979: 55). We felt that we had to make some attempt to investigate these matters, if only pragmatically, descriptively, and on a surface level, since, as the Select Committee pointed out, people caught in marital violence may 'need to consult with several different professionals in different places, employed by different agencies, very often not relating together very effectively' (Select Committee on Violence in Marriage 1975: para. 20).

Solicitors

Social workers, health visitors, and general practitioners were asked how they saw the role of the solicitor in relation to marital problems generally. A number of points were made and the easiest way to code them was to subdivide them according to whether or not they took a favourable view – as can be seen in *Table 11(1)*. Most of the favourable comments arose from an appreciation that people need legal advice and representation. Other points were: solicitors can help women to be decisive and to leave if the violence looks like continuing: they can be supportive to bewildered and demoralized battered wives; they can restrain partners from being unduly vindictive to each other.

Table 11(1) *Practitioners' views of solicitors*

	Social workers (n = 50) %	Health visitors (n = 50) %	GPs (n = 50) %
Favourable	54	36	18
Unfavourable	24	18	28
Mixed	12	24	52
No reply/don't know	10	22	2

Most of the adverse criticism concerned the solicitors' partisan role. For example a social worker remarked that 'They won't be neutral. They'll take a case and support that person to the hilt. But they are not concerned with fairness and justice to the other party'. And a health visitor observed that: 'Once they get involved battle lines get drawn, out come the affidavits. Then you notice the clients start using lawyers' battle talk'.

Doctors, in particular, seemed to have reservations about solicitors, often remarking that they had little interest in reconciling the parties. Although their complaints no doubt have some basis in reality, we do not feel that we have fully fathomed the reasons for the cool and even suspicious attitudes which in general characterize the relationship between doctors and solicitors.

Local authority social workers

Ninety per cent of the solicitors in our sample reported having varying amounts of contact with social workers. Those who often represented juvenile delinquents in court and those who had built up a fairly extensive practice helping battered wives, had the most contact. All the health visitors reported contact with social workers. Twenty-two per cent reported seeing social workers more often than once a fortnight but 52 per cent said that meetings tended to be infrequent. Fifty-six per cent of the doctors said that they used the health visitor to liaise on their behalf with Social Services and therefore generally had only indirect contact with them.

All three groups saw the Social Services Department as being useful in cases where there was an emergency need for accommodation. But health visitors and general practitioners, particularly, were often strongly ambivalent and critical when they were asked to comment on the social workers' role in relation to marital problems. Three main themes emerged from their evidence: first, social workers were often considered too inexperienced and too young to deal competently with clients' marital problems. Here are two typical comments:

> 'The problem is so many are so young. Mothers are always saying to me "I didn't tell her – she doesn't look as if she knows anything about it".' (Health visitor)

> 'They're not much use – lots of pleasant but immature young girls who like case conferences, writing reports, and talking, but they seem to get very little done. Some are good but most have too much theory and not enough contact with people. It's a pity they're not older and more experienced. I'd make them all nurse for six months.' (Doctor)

Second, the Social Services Department was seen as too large, bureaucratic, and impersonal.

> 'They won't do things quickly enough – bureaucratic anonymity breeds irresponsibility.' (Health visitor)

> 'I find them distant and rather anonymous. They seem to do everything through case conferences which take too long and are held at the wrong time for us GPs. They're too bureaucratic and pass the buck too much. They've let us down a lot so I'm cynical about them and not inclined to bother with them unless they're statutorily involved.' (Doctor)

Third, social workers were thought not likely to show much interest in cases of marital violence unless there were children.

> 'They tend not to get involved unless there's real risk to children. Otherwise they say they've no time to help, even though they have much smaller caseloads than we have.' (Health visitor)

> 'Unless you get a definite case of injury to children I don't think they have much to offer the battered wife syndrome.' (Doctor)

Health visitors

Solicitors had very little contact with health visitors and not much to say about them. Many confused them with local authority social workers. By contrast doctors and social workers were very closely involved with them and stressed the importance of their liaison role.

By comparison with themselves, social workers saw health visitors as non-stigmatic, and in touch with a wider range of families. As one said:

'They are a good front line for us. They pick up a lot of difficulties and pass them on to us. Everyone knows a health visitor more or less so they have a passport into all families and their knowledge of them is very great. They have no stigma as there is unfortunately with us.'

Another remarked, 'The health visitor I work most closely with observes a lot, hears things on the grapevine and passes it all on to me'.

Social workers seemed to be particularly conscious of the similarities between health visiting and social work: 'Social work is very much part of their brief, but they are short of time, are very busy, caseloads of hundreds compared with our thirty or so and so they don't go in too deeply'. Another remarked:

'They are probably as well equipped as social workers, but they don't visit as intensively as we do. They are often more acceptable to the family. An experienced health visitor with rapport is as capable as we are about helping with social problems and offering practical suggestions.'

A whiff of professional rivalry emerged from the comments of those social workers who emphasized the differences between the two professions: 'They have a minimal social work role. They can mess up cases by becoming over-involved and some encourage too much dependency and others go in waving a heavy stick. Their correct role is preventive medicine'. Another remarked: 'We see situations very differently. They tend to panic over matters where we think there is no cause for worry'.

Few social workers saw health visitors as having the time or the expertise to work with strained marriages. Health visitors were expected to refer either to Marriage Guidance or to the Social Services Department if they encountered a marital problem.

All doctors were asked how they saw the health visitor's role in relation to patients' marital problems. Two themes emerged: first, they were seen as a valuable source of information for the GPs' own endeavours in this field. 'An understanding ear people will talk to. She can save me a lot of time. She can also spend a bit longer finding out about the problems in the home than we can. Very often unhappy wives will talk to her woman-to-woman over a cup of tea'. Second, doctors thought they had an important practical role with families with small children: 'She is very good where children are involved and the family is experiencing practical difficulties. She knows the right strings to pull with social security and the social services'. Despite generally favourable comments, few doctors saw a role for health visitors in working therapeutically with their patients' marital problems.

Doctors

Solicitors, social workers, and health visitors were asked how they saw the doctor's role in relation to patients' marital problems. Their views were very mixed. GPs were seen to be in the best position to deal with these problems but their interest and response were thought to vary considerably.

> 'I find them a very mixed bunch, some helpful and some downright unhelpful. I had one case where a doctor told my client "Don't be so stupid. You married him, go back to him". I advised her to change her GP.' (Solicitor)

> 'I've five doctors I work to. They are all very different about this. Two are particularly good about counselling. The others are apt to rush to prescribe sedatives; they are factory-type doctors. They think there is nothing wrong if it's not physical.' (Health visitor)

> 'It depends on the doctor. A lot in my experience don't know much about mental health. Those who do are good and take time to discuss people's problems. Others just slap the pills in. They do not refer or counsel their patient and ignore the early warnings. Then we pick up the cases later which have been on valium for two years or more and who then say "I can't cope without my drugs"; cases which are much more difficult to help by then.' (Social worker)

Many health visitors and social workers were irritated with doctors who limited themselves to prescribing drugs.

Marriage Guidance

Solicitors, social workers, health visitors, and doctors were asked whether they had ever had any dealings with Marriage Guidance and whether they had any comments about it. *Table 11(2)* summarizes their replies.

The amount of contact reported is relatively high. Social workers had markedly less than the other practitioners. This may be because, on average, they had spent less time in post than the other practitioners. Adverse criticism greatly exceeded favourable comment. Even those in favour, mostly doctors, seemed more often impressed

Table 11(2) *Practitioners' response to Marriage Guidance*

	Solicitors (n = 50) %	Social workers (n = 50) %	Health visitors (n = 50) %	GPs (n = 50) %	Total (n = 200) %
No contact	18	38	16	8	20
Do use – favourable view	2	10	2	22	9
Some contact – no comment	46	4	54	12	29
Some contact – critical	34	46	28	58	41.5
No response	–	2	–	–	0.5

by the service's objectives than by its results. A number of practitioners drew attention to people's reluctance to use the service:

'I try to push it. I'm amazed how few people end up going. Perhaps by the time they get to a solicitor they know they want a divorce.' (Solicitor)

'There's something about MG. They'll only go when they are past it, and then the man won't usually go. It's rather like treating alcoholics – a lot depends on motivation and it's impossible to persuade some to go. Treatment is needed in the early stages but then they won't contemplate help. Once it's acknowledged it's often too late.' (Doctor)

We classify the many unfavourable opinions we received under the following headings, illustrating them with typical comments:

Middle-class/intellectual image

'Their way of working is possibly appropriate to the more intelligent customer. Our counselling in this practice is more directive, more practical advice, possibly because we have less time.' (Doctor)

> 'Clients of our type won't go. The counsellors are too upper crust, all twinset and pearls. It's OK for middle-class people whose marriages are going gently wrong. It's not relevant to women around here who are being severely battered.' (Health visitor)

'We can do just as well'

> 'If a patient can unburden himself to a GP he probably wouldn't get much more from MG. The common-sense ones we deal with; the more difficult cases need really skilled professional work. I have referred but then they pass them on to the psychiatric out-patient clinic and Professor —— who passes them back to me!' (Doctor)

Waiting lists cause delays

> 'The problem I've had is that I can never get an appointment in under three months. They seem to have a long waiting list. When things have cooled down a bit they don't want to go.' (Social worker)

No feedback

> 'A counsellor comes to this health centre each week. I suggest patients contact her but I never get any feedback.' (Doctor)

Does more good to counsellors than clients

> 'Dubious how much good it is. Counsellors get a good deal out of counselling – as much as their subjects.' (Doctor)

> 'I don't find them of much value. When you know counsellors and know about their own lives you wonder how they got the job.' (Doctor)

Ineffective

> 'I have referred – and they are some help. But I'm gradually coming to the conclusion that if one partner has made up his mind it's over, the marriage breaks up any rate. They may smooth things over for a while but the marriages break up in the end.' (Doctor)

Inappropriate to marital violence

'They can be very helpful but by the time things have got to the violent stage will you ever get the patients together? If good will isn't there, where parties can't make a go of it, counselling won't do it.' (Doctor)

Wrong method

'An awful lot of people don't feel they can take the physical step of going to MG. It's a real drawback that they don't visit people's homes as we do. Also a lot of our clients are asking for direction. They find it very difficult to grasp that what MG is doing is making them think about their situation.' (Social worker)

Too limited an approach

'Helpful where it's a situation of just husband and wife. It seems difficult for them if children are also involved. They don't seem well versed in that area.' (Social worker)

COMMENT

The extent of the adverse criticism that practitioners levelled at Marriage Guidance took us completely by surprise. The depth of their disenchantment was all too plain to see. It may be that Marriage Guidance has become a focus for the frustrations that other practitioners feel when dealing with intractable marital problems. This may be because Marriage Guidance is thought to be failing in its claim to be expert in the treatment of unhappy marriage. All four practitioner groups thought that while they themselves had the capacity to help less disturbed marital partnerships, Marriage Guidance should be able to deal with the difficult ones. The frustrations that fuelled many of their criticisms seemed to spring from a sense that as generalists they were being left to cope as best they could with large numbers of difficult cases including those where violence erupts dangerously.

Women's Aid

All practitioners were asked whether they had had direct contact with Women's Aid and the refuges they run and, if so, what they thought about them. *Table 11(3)* summarizes their replies.

Table 11(3) *Practitioners' response to women's refuges*

	Solicitors (n = 50) %	Social workers (n = 50) %	Health visitors (n = 50) %	GPs (n = 50) %	Total (n = 200) %
No contact	52	8	44	40	36.0
Contact – favourable	10	72	6	14	25.5
Contact – use very little/mixed/no comment	22	–	34	10	16.5
Contact – unfavourable	–	20	14	10	11.0
Did not know there was one	16	–	–	26	10.5
No reply	–	–	2	–	0.5

There were clear differences in attitude between the social workers on the one hand and the health visitors and doctors on the other. Social workers favoured refuges primarily because they provided them with an emergency back-up service for women in need of accommodation. Without them, social workers would face a desperately difficult problem.

Health visitors and doctors viewed refuges in a rather different light. Since they are called upon to visit in order to keep an eye on children or deal with sickness, they were most concerned with the overcrowding and poor physical conditions that generally pertain. Thus one doctor said:

> 'They are a good idea. There are two near here. But they haven't worked very well. They are trying hard but are short of funds. They tend to be overcrowded and look like slums. Putting all the women together creates an hysterical situation. They oughtn't to be lumped together like that. It's bad for the children.'

A health visitor remarked: 'I am supposed to liaise with them, but no one tells me when someone moves in. They are poorly organized. There's no staff there for the women to talk to or to help them. They are left to their own devices'.

Most of the doctors in our sample were men. Some disliked what they saw as the ardent feminism of the refuge organizers: 'I have quite a bit of contact. I need to call there. I have a feeling there are some Women's Lib people behind it. They turn a single domestic battle into gang warfare. They scare me stiff. They are chauvinistic in their own way'. Our impression was that despite such reservations, most practitioners welcomed the provision of refuges and thought there was a need to improve the quality of the services they provided. The prevailing view can be summarized by one of the social workers, who said: 'Refuges are absolutely essential. It's a superb idea but they have to work in such adverse circumstances and face so many obstacles that it's bound to be a bit rough and ready'. Nevertheless, many practitioners knew very little about refuges, probably because they are providing a service that has yet to establish itself in the public consciousness. The ignorance and ambivalence that practitioners revealed in relation to marital violence in general could be said to extend to the one specialist service that is trying to do something practical about the problem.

Discussion

Undercurrents of rival professional status and inter-group psychology infused and coloured many of the practitioners' comments about the role of other services dealing with marital problems. The status that practitioners give themselves, and have accorded to them, affects the way they relate to, and communicate with, other practitioners who may be seen as superior, equal, or inferior. For example, while many health visitors accepted that doctors had superior status, others complained that this denied them their rightful authority. Correspondingly, many doctors saw health visitors as aides, with lower status than themselves in the primary health care team. Broadly speaking, high status was accorded to those practitioners who took individual responsibility for their professional decisions. In this sense, solicitors and doctors were distinguished from the more bureaucratic social workers and health visitors. Our hierarchical culture has developed different communication patterns, which depend upon whether the communication is between perceived equals, or between superiors and inferiors, and vice versa. Deference is often a feature of the latter and was exemplified in many of the things the health visitors told us about their communication with doctors.

Differences in gender, marital status, and age are also involved in evaluating status. For example, the rather patronizing condescension shown by some male doctors to female health visitors may, in part, reflect traditional male paternalism towards women. We also noted that many of the older, married health visitors commented disparagingly on the youthful inexperience of single, female social workers.

All communication involves the problems of crossing boundaries. Our medical, legal, and social care systems may be conceived of as three distinct worlds, each with a different specialist language and set of professional values. In addition, each contains a complex network of related occupations. For example, the legal system contains barristers, solicitors, judges, court staff, etc., and the medical world contains doctors of various kinds, nurses, health visitors, medical psychologists, and so on. We have found it useful to think of frontiers that separate systems, and of boundaries that distinguish one occupational group from another within a given system. Thus, some forms of communication, for example between doctors and health visitors, merely involve crossing a boundary, whereas others, for example between doctors and solicitors, involve crossing frontiers. The latter are likely to be more difficult and complicated than the former, partly because the professional languages spoken on either side of the frontier are so different. In this respect it is worth noting that the health visitor has developed a specialist liaison role, crossing the frontier between medicine and social work, and very often acting as the GP's go-between in this respect. By taking on such a role she has to speak the languages of medicine and social work. By coming to rely on her for this task, the doctor may accord her more status and authority. At the same time, such a role may relieve the doctor of the task of developing skills to cross that frontier and may thus broaden the gulf between GPs and Social Services Departments.

New services, such as Women's Aid, face a particular problem in that they have to carve out territory for themselves. In so doing, their precise location in the network of services may not be clear to established practitioners in law, medicine, and social work. Sadly, it takes a long time for a new service to gain recognition for its own occupational ethos, for its language to be understood, and for its credibility to be secured. By contrast, Marriage Guidance represents an established organization whose tasks and methods, as well as achievements and limitations, are considered well understood, although this may not in fact be the case. Thus, a well-known voluntary organization like Marriage Guidance may have particular difficulty in convincing a professional audience that it has the capacity to adapt and improve its mode of work. Images stick, even though they may no longer be deserved.

All these matters are complicated and rather shadowy but they must affect the response of the practitioner to the client. Nevertheless, clients with marital problems are unlikely to have any idea how these factors influence practitioners who are working on their behalf, and who may ideally need to draw upon the resources of other services.

PART III

In Part II we examined factors that influence practitioners' individual responses to cases of marital violence. Now we shall widen our focus to consider the policy implications of victims' pattern of help-seeking during the various stages of marriage breakdown, and to discuss the important dynamic, but conflicting, contemporary influences determining the evolution of social policy. Finally, we argue that just as practices employed in dealing with individual cases determine the continuance or cessation of marital violence, so also will the character of our future policy influence the community's acceptance or rejection of it.

12
The significance of agency choice

Introduction

In 1977, when we began our investigation, there was virtually no published information to indicate what sort of people went to which particular service with what kind of marital problem. Divorce research has since shown that lawyers come into the picture usually only when one or both of the partners has decided that the relationship has broken down. By contrast, doctors seemed to be approached in the earlier stages of marital tensions.

We assume that people are most likely to go to services that they think will best meet their needs. Much therefore hinges on what they perceive these to be. This will depend on understanding their own circumstances, their knowledge of available resources, and their priorities. If they think of their problem in medical terms they will go to the doctor, if in legal terms to a solicitor, if in terms of accommodation to the housing department or social services, and so on. Very often, of course, they are conscious of having a variety of needs and are confused about which should have priority and where to go for particular help.

There is a further complication. The client's perception of need has to accommodate sufficiently well with the practitioner's if some course of action acceptable to both is to follow. Sometimes practitioners accept at face value what the clients tell them, but very often they make their own judgement about need. The meeting between a client and a practitioner thus often starts with some kind of negotiation about the client's needs. As we have argued, this is a tricky business for the practitioner, since it depends first on obtaining all the relevant and accurate information about the client's circumstances; second on the application of relevant professional knowledge; and third on the practitioner being conscious of his or her own professional and personal values and prejudices.

In addition to agency-specific needs, clients usually require social and emotional support; a sense that the practitioner has authority and competence; that he or she respects their privacy and treats them fairly. These are broad and rather ill-defined categories, but in our opinion they are as much key determinants of agency choice as the agency's function itself.

At this point we need to clarify what we mean by fair treatment. First, we use it to indicate the clients' subjective feelings that they have been given their due by public authorities. What is meant by giving someone their due is a complicated but ancient idea (Moyle 1912: 97).[1] It is concerned with the way people apply notions of justice to their personal relationships. It incorporates people's need for respect and is clearly linked with notions of identity and self esteem. Until quite recently the subject had not received much attention from the behavioural and social scientists (Walster, Walster, and Berscheid 1978; Boszormenyi-Nagy and Sparkes 1973), but it has a bearing on exchange in social relationships, as Homans (1961) recognized.

Second, in the context of dispute, fair treatment suggests a need to be dealt with in an impartial, even-handed way. In the study of divorcing couples to which we referred earlier, it was observed that:

> 'Curiously, even parents involved in the most acrimonious conflict seemed to retain a sense of an elusive middle ground between them which, with skill and understanding, could be identified by someone who was fair and impartial. It seems as if many people in conflict realize that the perceptions of each other have become in some way distorted, and often welcome the agency of concerned outsiders in their attempts to correct that distortion.' (Murch 1980: 173)

The needs for partisan support and neutral help appear to co-exist within the person. They do not necessarily pull in different directions. Simon Roberts, a legal anthropologist, has observed that where third parties align themselves in support of one or other of the disputants, 'while the strength of the respective sides may be altered, the fundamental bilateral character of the encounter remains unchanged' (Roberts 1979: 69). But when a third party seeks a neutral intermediary position and the disputants accept the authority of that position, the social structure of the conflict-resolving machinery alters fundamentally. The assumption the disputants make is that the intermediary will resolve the matter in an even-handed way acceptable to both sides. In overt marital disputes, particularly those that end in divorce, the need for partisan support may be uppermost in people's minds when they first seek help. By contrast it may be that people, anxious to improve their marriage, will seek neutral authority and fight shy of partisans. Whatever the case, as we have seen, many practitioners find it hard not to be partisan, although many feel uneasy about the unmet need for intermediary help.

The pattern of help-seeking

Other studies of marital violence indicate that there is a discernible pattern to the victim's search for help as the marital relationship deteriorates. Thus Pahl (1981), who interviewed forty-two women who used the Canterbury Refuge, showed that 'none of the women turned immediately to the helping professions on the first occasion on which violence occurred. For most the first reaction was one of shame and a sense of failure'.

Initially, many women feel unable to talk to anyone about the violence. If eventually they do, it is most likely to be to a friend or a member of the family. Pahl has written:

'Characteristically women turn to informal sources of help before formal sources of help and seek solutions which enable them to stay in their own homes before accepting solutions which involve them in leaving home.'

She concluded that

'it seems likely that the great majority of battered women either put up with the violence or find some solution to their problems without seeking the help of any professional except that of the solicitor who handles their divorce.'

The Dobashes (1980) found likewise. Of the 109 women they interviewed more than half talked to no-one after the first assault. But as violence continued, the chances of a woman seeking help from formal agencies, such as doctors, police, and social workers, increased. They point to a tendency for women to seek help or consolation 'without making their private problem any more public than necessary'. Binney, Harkell, and Nixon (1981) found that of 636 women they interviewed from refuges, the average number of agencies or individuals from whom they had sought help was five. Surprisingly, they also discovered that the average number of agencies contacted remained the same no matter how long a woman had suffered violence. They suggested that 'repeated failure to gain the type of help needed left women feeling demoralized'. The implication is that if appropriate help is not found early the woman tends to give up the search for it until there is an emergency.

The progression in the normal pattern of help-seeking, from informal support from friends and relatives, on to seeking support from doctors or social workers, and then eventually to lawyers and to law enforcement agencies such as the police, carries with it a progressive risk of loss of privacy. Criminal prosecution of aggressive partners takes place under the full glare of press reporting where the identity of the victim may be revealed to all. As in the case of rape, the prospect of going to court may well deter many victims from seeking help in the first place. We surmise that, as a general rule, it is only when the conflict in domestic partnerships is felt by one or both to be getting dangerously out of control, that help is likely to be sought from an agency of social control such as the police, in the hope that the aggressive partner will be challenged, restrained, even punished.

Early stages of marriage breakdown

THE GENERAL PRACTITIONER

When a deteriorating domestic relationship, possibly accompanied by violence, reaches the point where one or even both partners feels driven to seek help beyond their immediate circle of friends and relatives, they are most likely to turn to their GP (Chester 1973; Murch 1975; Pahl 1981; Mitchell 1981). Divorce studies (Murch 1975; Mitchell 1981) show that women are approximately twice as likely as men to consult their doctor about marital problems, but they are often very ambivalent about it. They may feel ashamed, uncertain about the kind of reception to expect, and worried about losing face. They may feel they are being disloyal to their partner and that they should be coping with their own problems.

Although medical symptoms such as headaches, sleeping difficulties, and depression, may justify a visit to the doctor, people may turn to their doctor for other reasons. Women usually already have an established relationship with their doctor, particularly if he or she has been involved in their pre-natal care. Most trust the doctor to respect confidentiality and there is no stigma involved in going to surgery. Culturally, the doctor is often perceived as a symbolic authority figure. Since the GP is often seen as the 'family' doctor, many patients expect that their doctor will retain impartial concern extending to their partner and children as well. This may be particularly important in the early stages of marriage breakdown when the patient herself still has a commitment to keeping the family and the marriage together. If she is worried about losing face by overtly acknowledging her marital difficulties, a perceptive doctor may protect her self-esteem by treating her medical symptoms while appreciating the underlying relationship difficulties. She is thus able to maintain a semblance to the outside world that her marriage is functioning 'normally'.

Tragically, as we have seen, only half the GPs we interviewed considered it 'real medicine' to be concerned with their patients' marital problems. The remainder stuck to an orthodox view, defining marital tensions and violence as social rather than medical. Other researchers (Byrne and Long 1976; Pahl 1979) have described how patients report that such doctors do not encourage them to talk and usually dismiss them quickly with a prescription for valium. Our interviews with health visitors confirmed this. A basic change of attitude by these doctors is required so that they at least acknowledge that marital problems are an important area of family medicine. Part of the problem may be that GPs do not appreciate that they are the key agency of first instance in the early stages of marriage breakdown. The Royal College of General Practitioners and the Department of Health and Social Security ought, in our opinion, to impress this upon doctors and help them to develop appropriate skills through professional and post-professional education.

The standard surgery appointment time is less than ten minutes. When the waiting room is crowded the doctor is inevitably under pressure to hurry cases through. However perceptive the doctor might be, this does not give an ambivalent woman adequate time to explain her story. Some doctors try to overcome this by asking patients to come back after surgery. It might well help if one partner in group practices took special responsibility for the treatment of marital problems, taking referrals from the other partners. Ideally, doctors ought to have more time for the initial consultation so that neither they nor their patients should feel inhibited from gently exploring these sensitive, personal problems. But we recognize that it is difficult to reorganize the standard pattern of surgery appointments to allow this to happen.

More might be done to establish better working partnerships between doctors and health visitors. Health visitors are in a good position to offer support and information to wives, while the doctor has the necessary authority to challenge domineering and violent husbands. The scope of the health visitors' responsibilities should be widened so that they should be available at the request of the GP to help any women who are experiencing marital violence, not just those with small children. Health visitors should be able to give victims some clear information about their welfare and legal entitlements, advice on how to use other services, and where to find emergency accommodation if violence is a feature of the relationship.

One disadvantage of a policy seeking to extend the responsibilities of GPs and health visitors is that it might perpetuate a belief that marital problems are to be defined primarily in terms of illness. Many would disagree with this. The Dobashes (1980) for example, who take a strong feminist view, have pointed out that the medical model of disease 'deflects the focus from the historically established authority relationships between men and women to personal explanation'. They would argue that a conservative and largely male-dominated profession such as medicine is culturally bound to accept the 'rightful authority' of patriarchy in family relations. In our view this is not an argument against developing the GPs' responsibility in this field – consumer choice is dictating that. Rather, it supports the case for educating the medical profession about the nature and causes of marital violence and for broadening their understanding.

MARRIAGE GUIDANCE

The traditional role of Marriage Guidance is thrown into question if one accepts that GPs are pre-eminently the agency of first choice in dealing with deteriorating marriages. Despite all the effort and public resources that have been put into Marriage Guidance since the War, and the training and expertise that has been built up, Marriage Guidance has only been able to attract what is by comparison with the number of divorces and strained marriages a mere handful of clients. The Home Office Working Party on Marriage Guidance explains this by saying that 'many people are reluctant to admit to having difficulties in marriage and find it hard to believe that anything can be done' (Home Office Working Party on Marriage Guidance 1979: 25). The large number of people seeking help from doctors tends to belie this. But the evidence does suggest that many people fight shy of taking their marital problems *overtly* to strangers. Yet Marriage Guidance almost demands this of their clients. Moreover, our investigation about practitioners' views of this service suggests it has a poor image which may further account for the relatively low referral rate. Binney, Harkell, and Nixon (1981) found that the women they interviewed in refuges counted Marriage Guidance amongst the least helpful of all the public services available.

It may well be that potential clients are put off by an approach that encourages them to find the answers by examining their own behaviour and motivations from a new perspective. While this may be all very well for a limited number of people who are capable of such insights into the management of conflict, there are probably many more for whom it is inappropriate, at least when under a lot of stress. At that time people first and foremost need sympathetic partisan support, although additional help from neutral conciliators may be acceptable as well. Merely relying on a counselling approach that requires people to examine their own unconscious collusions with their partners and to search for strength within themselves may be baffling and demoralizing.

We think the work of Marriage Guidance should be gradually absorbed into the health service and become a specialist back-up resource for GPs. For example, Marriage Guidance might take the initiative, in collaboration with the Department of Health and Social Security, in setting up marital training and development groups along the lines suggested by the Home Office Working Party on Marriage Guidance (1979). These groups would be able to offer valuable consultation to the primary health care team, helping them to develop their skills by in-service training. If some of the organization problems revealed by experiments in this field could be overcome, more might also be done in attaching experienced Marriage Guidance counsellors to GPs' surgeries. From a policy formulation point of view, the fact that Marriage Guidance receives a substantial proportion of its funding from the Home Office rather than the Department of Health and Social Security, might hamper such a move into the Health Service. Moreover, Marriage Guidance, as a well-established organization, may have strong motivation to preserve its distinct identity by resisting such a development. However, in so doing it may unwittingly collude with society's tendency to make merely token provision for the huge numbers of people experiencing marital problems.

LOCAL AUTHORITY SOCIAL SERVICES

It could be argued that it would be more feasible to develop local authority social services than to improve the GP service or breathe new life into Marriage Guidance. Since the War, social work has shown a remarkable facility for extending the range and nature of its responsibilities. Local authority social workers have smaller caseloads than doctors and health visitors; their training gives them a knowledge of community services, and some are undoubtedly skilled enough to work intensively with people experiencing marital problems. Nevertheless, the evidence suggests that the public are not much inclined to take their marital problems to Social Services Departments (Mattinson and Sinclair 1979). The reasons for this are clear. As with Marriage Guidance, the onus is put on clients to declare overtly the existence of marital problems to a stranger. Moreover, as we have seen, there is evidence (Murch 1980) to suggest that these Departments are regarded by their clientele as stigmatic. Various researchers (George and Wilding 1972; Mitchell 1981; Pahl 1981) have shown that potential clients are deterred from approaching these Departments because they believe that rather than being offered direct practical help they will be covertly supervised, their children placed on 'at risk' registers or even removed into care. Pahl reports some cases where 'husbands used this power as a threat, telling their wives that a breakdown within the family would result in the removal of children' (1981: 71). Furthermore, as we have seen, many practitioners in other services regard social workers as too often young and lacking in professional and life experience, a view often shared by clients (Murch 1980). Our analysis of the respective age and length of experience of our four practitioner groups shows that there is factual evidence to support this view (see Appendix). Many social workers also seem doubtful about their contribution to this field. When their primary responsibility is to children, they can be in a difficult position when faced with clients' marital problems because, in a violent, stress-filled home, the needs of individuals often pull in opposite directions. For these reasons, and given the ambiguities in the social workers' role to which we referred earlier, we think it would be placing an unnecessary burden upon them to expect them to provide a major service to people with marital problems.

Termination of marriage:
the changing pattern of help-seeking

SOLICITORS

When the domestic relationship deteriorates to the point that one or other of the parties feels that escape from the tensions is necessary, an

The significance of agency choice 191

approach to a lawyer is usually made. Contrary to popular opinion, the great majority of those who divorce have already made up their mind to do so before consulting a solicitor (Dobash 1980; Murch 1980). Notwithstanding the withdrawal of Legal Aid from undefended divorce, 99 per cent of divorce petitioners still turn to a solicitor when their marriage breaks down (Davis, Macleod, and Murch 1982), often receiving advice and assistance under the so-called Green Form Scheme. Studies of the divorcing population in Scotland (Mitchell 1981) and in England and Wales (Murch 1980) have shown that the overwhelming majority of clients were satisfied with their solicitors' services, largely because they provide partisan support as well as legal advice. Like GPs, they are also regarded as non-stigmatic.

It is clearly important that solicitors have enough time to explore thoroughly the nature of their clients' problems when they first interview them. It ought to be remembered that the amount of time available is determined by the level of remuneration that solicitors receive. Attempts to restrict the provision of Legal Aid and advice may therefore dilute the quality and usefulness of their service.

CONCILIATION SERVICES

In 1974, the Finer Committee drew attention to the fragmented court structure for dealing with family matters and argued that it was too expensive and adversarial in character. They suggested a unified system of family courts and procedures to encourage easier settlement of family differences by negotiation and conciliation. Since then, although very little progress has been made to implement the Finer Committee's proposals, local initiatives have been taken to establish conciliation services. In 1982 the Government set up an Inter-Departmental Committee on conciliation, comprising officials from the Lord Chancellor's Department, the Home Office, the Department of Health and Social Security, the Central Policy Review Staff, and the Treasury, with terms of reference to report to Ministers on the nature, scope, and effects of conciliation services and to consider whether, and if so how, they should be promoted or developed. This Committee, which is due to report in the Spring of 1983, might possibly herald a major strategic policy change in the provision of legal and associated services to people with marital problems.

Where marital violence is concerned, some County Court judges believe that there is a case for making greater use of conciliation when injunctions are sought. They argue that since violence is often indicative of emotional attachments between the partners, conciliation, backed by the authority of the court, may restrain it. It may also help parties to a more rational solution of problems concerning the division of property and the care of children. Yet the Dobashes (1980) have argued that in those cases where violence is symptomatic of a man's dominance, attempts to provide impartial conciliation will be perceived by the woman as a failure to give her the support she needs – even as a reinforcement of the husband's position. Where the power of the parties is unequal, impartiality by outsiders does not correct the balance.

Emergency services

THE POLICE

At virtually any stage in a marriage, violence may erupt savagely so that the police are called. Practically all emergency cases reflect a demand for a powerful external authority to come in and take charge of things. Where marital violence is concerned, the primary need is for the aggressor to be restrained. But generally speaking, until the police are satisfied that an offence has occurred, they adopt a neutral stance. Many women, wanting the risk of further violence removed, report this to be of little help, considering the police to be tacitly agreeing with their husband.

As things stand at present, once the police have decided it is not a case for prosecution they withdraw from the scene, usually having calmed the situation (their very arrival may do that), and give a few words of advice about the kinds of social help that might be available. The result is that although control and possible help have arrived, they quickly vanish. Given other demands on police patrols this is understandable. The police often leave the scene rapidly, and this may well leave a woman in a continuing state of fear, feeling that having once asked for police help she cannot do so again. Little wonder that so many women in refuges later say 'the police just didn't want to know' (Jeffery and Pahl 1979). But such a response is often totally inadequate psychologically and emotionally and falls far short of what is required – namely the prospect of some continuing support and readily accessible control while the partners are working through a volatile and dangerous crisis.

The police themselves have pinpointed the difficulty. For example, in the evidence given by police organizations to the Parliamentary

The significance of agency choice   193

Select Committee on Violence in Marriage (1975), there appear the following remarks:

'It is a significant and rather a sad fact that the police are the only agency available twenty-four hours a day. It is almost impossible at times to get a Marriage Guidance counsellor or social worker out of office hours. I sometimes think it is easier for a camel to go through the eye of a needle than for this to happen. But quite often we can go to these domestic disputes and peace can descend and you fear something will flare up again once you go. But you cannot make an arrest because you have not got the grounds for doing so. If people were available on a twenty-four-hour basis, as the police are, we could then send for the social worker straight away.' (Evidence of Chief Superintendent Dow, para. 1591)

'I feel at the moment the police are spending a lot of time on something which is not really a police matter, when we go and there is no offence, but we have no-one else to channel the problem to at that particular time if it is out of office hours.' (Evidence of Chief Superintendent Keyte, para. 1592)

Clearly, some form of twenty-four-hour back-up is needed to take over from the police patrol as soon as the violence has been quelled. A way to meet this need must be found. One implication of Farragher's research (1981) is that it is possible to link up volunteers to police intervention in individual cases so that a volunteer arrives on the scene more or less when the police do. We think there are opportunities here for useful experiment. Another useful idea is the provision of an alarm system installed in the victim's home linked direct to the local police station. This would be particularly helpful in those cases where the parties are living apart and where the victim has already obtained an injunction for non-molestation, possibly with a power of arrest attached. We have heard of one such experiment in the North-East.

MEDICAL SERVICES

We turn now to emergency medical services. Since, proportionate to the number of cases going to hospital accident departments, those involving marital violence are few, it is clearly difficult for staff to be constantly on the lookout for them. Identifying cases is further complicated because some women keep quiet about the cause of their injuries. It should be remembered too that violence is not always directed at the other partner; it may be self-imposed. Morgan (1979) has shown that many cases of self-laceration or attempted suicide occur when the patient, usually a woman, has experienced a breakdown in her domestic relationship. But even where the hospital does know the cause of injury, often little is done to ensure that the patient is given after-care support. Many doctors to whom we spoke complained that they are not informed when their patients are treated in accident departments. Some patients might not want their GP to know and may even have sought hospital treatment to avoid him. On the other hand, we think some women would welcome help after discharge. Much depends on the ability of the hospital staff to identify cases and discuss with the patients the possibility of referral to the GP or health visitor. Whatever the case, we would like to see more effective communication between accident departments and the primary health care team.

EMERGENCY ACCOMMODATION: REFUGES

The need for emergency accommodation has only been highlighted since the women's movement began to establish and develop a network of refuges. The moment refuges were established they attracted a clientele. Why? Because they offered something practical and backed it with emotional commitment to the women concerned. Improving the quality of refuge provision and developing the range of related services would be an important way of encouraging such women to escape from violence. All the evidence suggests that they need protection, safe accommodation, an enormous amount of compassionate support, and encouragement as they rebuild their self-confidence. This may well be help of the kind best provided in the first instance by other women.

At present refuges face acute financial problems. This is partly because central government is not anxious to take on new welfare commitments and because many refuges only secured short-term funding in the 1970s under the Urban Aid scheme. Thus there is now a critical question: how to provide the necessary permanent finance for an adequate network of refuges? One can argue that a substantial proportion of their funds should come out of local authority Social Services budgets since it is clear that referral to refuges is a major part of the help social workers now give battered wives. On the other hand, there are strong arguments that refuges benefit from their independence from statutory services and from the ethos of self-help. The difficulty is that self-help organizations may not be particularly successful in capturing financial resource in times of recession. Because of this, we think the future of refuges now hangs in the balance. Those running them face important strategic political and ideological questions, which we discuss in the next chapter.

Court proceedings

We turn now to injunction procedure and criminal prosecution. Since we did not make a close study of the court proceedings we cannot base our conclusions on first-hand experience. But some solicitors, county court registrars, and judges have told us that occasionally an injunction is used as a tactical move in the battle over matrimonial property. If this is so, we deprecate the practice on the grounds that it can only serve to strain the relationship further, lead to a sense of injustice in the man, and possibly increase the risk of further violence. We have also been told that the practice of seeking emergency Legal Aid Certificates is open to abuse as a way of circumventing the shortcomings of the Green Form Scheme. These things should be investigated.

In the case of criminal prosecutions two serious procedural shortcomings stand out: the delay that often occurs in bringing proceedings; and the practice of allowing men to return home on bail. According to Jeffery and Pahl (1979), only a quarter of the cases studied had been concluded within three weeks of the offence, and 'final disposal of the cases could be as long as forty-seven weeks'. Such delays often place the couple in the appalling situation of having to continue to live together in the weeks leading up to the trial, both partners knowing that the evidence of one will support the prosecution of the other and possibly lead to a conviction resulting in imprisonment.

It is clearly wrong in these circumstances for the woman who fears further violence to feel that she is the one who has to leave the house and seek shelter elsewhere. Moving is expensive both emotionally and financially for women and children. It would be better if the man had somewhere else to go. The civil injunction procedure clearly helps in this respect, but in cases where criminal prosecution is pending, simultaneous civil proceedings for injunctions are not always used. It would help if, as a condition of bail, the man was ordered to live elsewhere.

Another obvious shortcoming of criminal proceedings lies in the nature of the penalties usually imposed by the courts. Jeffery's survey (1979) of 174 police records concerning criminal prosecution in cases of marital violence showed that only six resulted in a prison sentence. The most common penalty, occurring in 63 per cent of the convicted cases, was some form of 'binding over' to keep the peace. Most of the remainder were fined, the amounts ranging from £5 to £200. Curiously there is no mention of the use of probation in the study. Nevertheless, it is clear that in the majority of cases convicted men remain free, without any form of supervision, to pose a continuing threat to their wives. If a man is fined and resents it, the wife is the obvious scapegoat. Even if he refrains from further assault the tensions between the couple will probably be further strained. If the couple are separated and the man has an obligation to maintain, he may default on maintenance. Of course, we recognize that a probation order with conditions of residence or even a short prison sentence is not going to eliminate these difficulties altogether. But it would give women a respite from the pressure of living with a violent husband and a chance to take stock of the family's life and, if need be, do something about it. It could help the husband too.

Our basic unease is with the sentencing policy of the courts. We suspect that too often they regard assault arising from marital violence as somehow 'vaguely domestic' and therefore not serious crime. We think it likely that such a sentencing mentality fails to come to grips both with the element of criminality which needs punishment and the element of marital conflict that needs containment and help. That is why we find it strange that probation supervision is not often used. We strongly suspect that of all categories of offenders, men who assault their wives are most likely to respond to the traditional probation approach which seeks to advise, assist, and befriend.

Consumer choice

Before leaving the issue of agency choice, we should mention the related subject of the client's selection of individual worker. Generally speaking, except in the case of solicitors and possibly doctors, clients have very little chance to choose their practitioner. Even so, there is a fair amount of evidence to suggest that they do observe characteristics of practitioners and use them to estimate professional competence. Murch (1980) has shown that in the case of divorce court welfare officers people had most confidence in practitioners who were themselves married and had children of their own. They complained about social workers who were 'immature student types, all theory and little experience'.

The significance of agency choice 197

Apart from trying to assess professional competence in various ways, in our opinion the basic questions that people with marital problems usually ask themselves before going to a service are:

'Will I get a sympathetic supportive response?'
'Will the service be able to alter things for the better?'
'Will they treat my affairs in confidence?'
'Will they treat me fairly?'

These fundamental questions can be thought of as the variables of social support, privacy, social control, and fairness in approach, all of which influence the individual's decision to seek help.

Collaboration between services

If, as we suggest, clients make some kind of intuitive calculation of these variables, both in their initial choice of agency and, where feasible, in their choice of practitioner, and if as we also suggest, individual agency practice develops a particular organizational role-set in response to a combination of these variables (some offering primarily social and emotional support, others emphasizing social control, some paying stricter attention to confidentiality than others), then it follows that conscious attempts to promote collaboration and referral between services in individual cases are almost bound to distort the balance of factors which led to the *client's* initial choice. Professional collaboration can easily overlook this. Furthermore, it may also be that some practitioners weigh up similar considerations in deciding how far to collaborate with other services. For example, services that have a predominantly social control function may have difficulty working closely with those which do not; those that place a high premium on confidentiality will not work easily with those that do not; non-stigmatic services might fight shy of referring clients to services seen as stigmatic; partisans may be suspicious of intermediaries.

As we have already pointed out, the collaboration rhetoric in which practitioners and policy-makers frequently indulge[2] tends in our view to overlook these problems, and mask the way both consumers and practitioners discriminate between services and, indeed, clusters of services.

But while these ideas may explain incompatibilities, they may also, of course, identify those whose general characteristics predispose them towards good diplomatic relations, an idea that should be borne in mind when thinking about the direction that social policy should take. This point supports our general view that in the early stages of marriage breakdown the primary health care team should mainly provide the help, and that legal services, which operate with a very different professional ethos, should take over as the main source of assistance when relationships are finally breaking down.

Notes

1 The first book of Justinian's Institutes begins, 'Justitia est constans et perpetua voluntas ius suum cuique tribuens', translated as meaning, 'justice is the set and constant purpose which gives to everyman his due'.
2 See Home Office Working Party on Marriage Guidance 1979: 55. The Working Party states: 'Collaboration is vital to our concept of a network of services of different sorts attracting different groups of clients in varied ways'; 'Collaboration is never easy which presumably is why it is more talked about than practised'; 'It requires a great deal of work and time; there are no short cuts'.

13
Some policy considerations

Social values determine the definition of social problems, which in turn influence policies. A difficulty with marital violence is that it attracts a confusing amalgam of potentially conflicting values. It raises issues of individual responsibility and freedom, of justice and equality, and of loyalty and privacy in personal relationships. It is concerned with the values we ascribe to marriage, the family, the respective position of women, men, and children, and the relationship of all these to our industrial, mixed-economy society. It involves complex questions about power in personal relationships and about the circumstances in which power expressed as violence may be sanctioned. Value-judgements about all these matters influence people's views whether, and in what circumstances, the State should care for and protect victims of marital and family violence. As we have seen, they also affect people's perception of marital violence in the first place, how they define and explain it, and how they respond to it.

Retrenchment

Contemporary Government policy has become known in general terms as a policy of retrenchment rather than reform. Winkler (1981) has shown that retrenchment involves a general move to off-load the provision of services onto the local community:

> 'Across the whole range of social policy, recent British governments both Labour and Conservative, have been developing institutions for involving the "community" in the provision of welfare services. These developments are commonly presented as being better for the recipient, more cost-effective and, more grandly, a superior form of social organisation as well. Stripped of these rationals, however, in straightforward descriptive terms what the state has been doing is off-loading some of its hitherto accepted welfare obligations back onto its citizens.' (Winkler 1981: 82)

He explains that:

> 'The off-loading process thus consists of three linked operations, the transfer of existing services to the community, the pre-emption of demand, and the mobilization of new community provision. It is important to recognize that what is being off-loaded is not just statutory services, but obligations to deal with social problems.'
> (1981: 134)

To support his argument he points to the way such a policy has been pursued in a variety of services involving public expenditure – housing, health, general social services and education – all with the aim of reducing public expenditure and the financial problems of the Welfare State.[1]

If Winkler's analysis is correct, there are profound implications for the development of a social policy for marital violence. For example, it suggests that the best that can be hoped for is Government support for the relatively inexpensive piecemeal development of *existing* services rather than assuming *new* responsibilities for refuges, conciliation services attached to family courts, and so on. While the theory of retrenchment would support the self-help ethos underlying the provision of refuges by the women's groups, it would draw the line at financial support. It would favour the use of volunteers in advisory services such as Citizens' Advice Bureaux and Women's Aid rather than the extension of services employing fully trained professionals. Marriage Guidance would go on playing a token role, their very existence providing some sort of excuse for not developing the role of the GP despite the obvious consumer preference. The police would not be encouraged to improve the quality of their emergency services in domestic cases which might be given even lower priority than at present. Steps might be taken to reduce the level of expenditure on civil legal aid in matrimonial cases. The inadequacies of court procedures, to which we referred in the last chapter, would remain. There would be no further Government support for research. Moreover, those committed to improving the quality of services to deal with marital violence will be competing for dwindling Government funds with other interest groups seeking to find policy solutions to newly emerging problems such as mass unemployment, racial tension, and civil disorder. The basic implication of a retrenchment policy is that adults, families, and local communities should solve their own problems rather than bother the State with them.

Some policy considerations 201

Even if the goodwill and interest of Government can be sustained, staff cuts in the Civil Service and local government will result in fewer administrators with time available to develop and implement new policies; policies which in any event would require co-ordination in central government where departmental fragmentation interferes with an overall view of the subject.

Reformist ideologies

Given such a climate, how might social policy advance? Much will depend on the strength of the main ideologies committed to reform: child-saving, familism, feminism, and Marxism. At the risk of oversimplification, the essentials of their approach to marital violence may be summarized in the following way.

CHILD-SAVING

The child-centred approach has strong institutional support in social work and social medicine. It leads to policies that put strong emphasis on covert surveillance of families, preventive case work, and the rescuing of children perceived to be at risk. The idea that family violence, whether between parents or directed at the children, might increase the likelihood of the children growing up to be violent in adult life, provides the main justification for interventionist policies that reflect this approach. Pizzey gave credence to such a view when, in her evidence to the Select Committee, she said 'I believe that many of the children born into violence grow up to be aggressive psychopaths, and it is the wives of such men that we see at Chiswick' (Select Committee on Violence in Marriage 1975: 2). One consequence of this view is a refusal to offer help to battered wives unless they are the mothers of young children. We encountered this attitude in our interviews with some social workers and health visitors, and it may also underlie a recent suggestion that the Department of Health and Social Security should only be concerned with refuges in so far as they are seen as providing a form of residential care for children.

FAMILISM

In general, familists are particularly concerned with the stresses and strains on families that erupt into violence. Thus, they favour policies aimed at reducing stress and reinforcing family solidarity. Although they often find common cause with child-savers, they have a greater tendency to focus on the interests of the family as a whole rather than on the welfare of children or individual adults. They tend to see the family as the key social unit of society, a view that emerges, for example, in a recent report of a sub-committee of the Society of Conservative Lawyers which asserted that:

> 'The family is the foundation of our free democratic society. For the great majority of people in Britain, the family is formed by the institution of marriage which is a union for life and is the vital link which binds the family. A stable family life within the bonds of matrimony is still the popular ideal. If there is a failure to live up to that ideal, if marriages break down or are unstable, then the whole of society is weakened. The State is therefore vitally concerned in the preservation of marriages, and when there are children, vitally concerned to preserve a stable two-parent family united in marriage.' (Society of Conservative Lawyers 1981: 11)

Donzelot (1980) has shown that in our Western society familism is of fairly recent origin, and developed strongly in the last century. He suggests that it grew as a consequence of industrialization and that in post-war years it has received powerful ideological reinforcement from psychoanalysis. Certainly, in our study we could detect in many of our interviews with social workers, health visitors, and doctors the undercurrents of these modes of thought. They sometimes seemed to contribute to a certain scepticism about the women's movement, as if feminism was seen as undermining the stability of family life by attacking the role of mothers within it.

FEMINISM

Where marital violence is concerned, feminism has spearheaded almost all the advances of the last decade, including the network of refuges. With a simple, direct, intellectually plausible message, it has a broad and powerful constituency. From the feminist perspective held by many women who run refuges, marital violence is seen as symptomatic of a patriarchal culture. For them, refuges symbolize more than philanthropic provision for oppressed and frightened women. Thus the Dobashes have advanced the view that refuges

> 'represent a symbolic acknowledgement of the legitimacy of the activities and concerns of women and a rejection of male violence.

To the agencies, they stand as an illustration that direct and pragmatic support is workable and beneficial, albeit not without its problems. To the violent husband, they are a pragmatic denial of the assumption that a man's wife is a possession who can be treated with relative impunity because it is difficult for her to escape from his dominion. The overall significance of the (Women's) Federation's response to wife beating is its combination of the strength of female culture (supporting women and rejecting male abuses) with feminist principles that locate these abuses in the subordinate status of women. There is unequivocal rejection of the man's right to use violence against his wife, and a challenge to the patriarchal assumptions and relationships that so long supported that right.' (Dobash and Dobash 1981: 575-76)

MARXISM

Two writers have recently suggested that a Marxist analysis might add something to the feminist perspective and throw more light on the causes of marital violence and on the direction that social policy should take. Leonard and McLeod argued that feminism does not sufficiently relate itself conceptually to the political and economic structure:

'We need to know what sustains and reproduces patriarchy at an ideological and material level, and how this penetrates and moulds the experiences of those involved in marital violence. Much work needs to be done to articulate the relationship between the concept of a patriarchal social order, the means by which production and social reproduction takes place in society, and the connection with social interaction within the family.' (Leonard and McLeod 1980: 9)

Work of this kind might, for example, explore the way the profit motive in industry uses images of masculine dominance and physical prowess in commercial promotion, for example, of alcohol, commonly believed to be associated with violence. In another paper, Leonard (1981), whose research involved interviews with male assailants, suggested that frustrations which men experience in their work might encourage them to displace aggression onto their wives.

Ideological conflict

The protagonists of child-saving, familism, feminism, and Marxism cannot agree the prime causes of marital violence. Different causes suggest different solutions. Each wants to put the emphasis of social policy in a rather different place. For example, the feminists' aim of freeing women from what they see as the culture-bound, subordinate roles of wife within marriage and mother within family clearly conflicts with the view of child-savers and familists who believe these roles should be reinforced wherever possible. The feminists' challenge to familism is well illustrated in the following comments taken from a document prepared by a Women's Aid Federation research group:

'There is little or no appreciation of the mental and emotional suffering created by a society that recognizes and values women only for their service to men and as good mothers. This devaluation of women as persons in their own right adds to the experience of battering, the stigma of failure. We should look again at the responsibility for children which women assume, and which society expects of them, especially in the creation and maintenance of dependency of women on men. Dependency is the most powerful factor in keeping women within a violent situation, in taking them back there, and in preventing the development of the independence of women.' (Women's Aid Federation 1981)

Our concern is that policy-makers in central government can, and probably will, use the lack of agreement about the nature of the problem as an excuse for inaction. Indeed, there is a danger that the more explicit the differing reformist ideologies become, the more difficult it will be to find even a minimal degree of consensus between them. This may explain the inaction on the part of the DHSS following the conference that they organized in Canterbury in September 1981. The discussion at that conference highlighted dramatically some of the competing ideologies. Ann Shearer pointed out in *The Guardian* (September 1981) that a number of professionals, including social workers, health visitors, and the DHSS's own Research Liaison Group reacted defensively to what she termed 'the insistent arguments of the radical feminists of Women's Aid'. In Shearer's view, Women's Aid were demanding a revolution in the attitudes of professional care-givers.

After the conference, an authoritative source within the DHSS told us that the DHSS was changing its view about the 'correct' definition of the problem of marital violence. We were told that when the Department initially sponsored research in 1977, following the recommendations of the Select Committee, they were more inclined to share the view of the women's movement that violence should be understood primarily in terms of sexual politics and patriarchy. After the conference, those sections of the DHSS concerned with the development of services for children and families evidently became more aware that the feminists' viewpoint represented something of a doctrinal challenge to their interests, which in any event were being threatened from other directions by economic cuts and the policy of retrenchment.

So by 1982 efforts to involve central government in policy development had run into a depressing impasse. As far as we have been able to discover, the Government does not propose to develop a social policy. It appears to have no plans to finance refuges in the long term or to help practitioners in the health and social services become more aware of the problem or to commission further research.

In these circumstances, it seems to us that if any progress towards a coherent policy is to be made, some common ground must be found between feminists and professional care-givers to bridge the gaps that are opening between them.

Social justice

All of them, in different ways, are fighting against some form of perceived oppression – the oppression of children by negligent parents, the social oppression of disadvantaged families, the oppression of women by men, or even the oppression of the poor by the rich. They share a common belief that oppression undermines human dignity. The justice they seek is generally of a distributive rather than of a retributive kind, in the sense that each ideology is trying to give a stronger voice to the weak in the struggle against the powerful. In the case of family violence that struggle sometimes turns into a struggle for life itself since, in its extreme form, violence results in homicide.

Familists, child-savers, and feminists have already done much to bring family violence into public consciousness. In that sense, more by luck than judgement, they have already taken common cause to good effect. The complexities of the subject are being identified and slowly unravelled. New forms of provision are being thought about and developed. But in the future, the imponderable question is whether the supporters of these ideologies will see themselves as part of a wider movement for social justice or whether their emotional commitment to doctrine will force each to fight the other in the struggle for scarce resources. If that happens, the danger is that public attention will be diverted from the continuing need to hammer out fair and practical policies for victims of family violence, whether they be children or adults. In our opinion this would represent yet another form of collusion with the community's long-standing tendency to deny the realities of the problem. Ideological debate would then be seen merely as flight into objectivity and the community would have failed to translate its growing understanding of the problem into anything of practical value.

Finally, just as practitioners' responses to individual cases may determine the continuance or cessation of marital violence, so also will the character of social policy influence the community's acceptance or rejection of it. Throughout five years' research we have been aware of a constant tendency both in practice and policy to shuffle away from a frank recognition that very large numbers of people are caught in miserable domestic relationships and experience violence that endangers their physical and emotional well-being. The scale of the problem may be far greater than anything suggested to the Select Committee. Thus, as we argued in Chapter 2, as many as one in five marriages may experience some violence. On current trends at least one in four marriages will end in divorce and many more will endure through periods of tension and unhappiness.

When one considers social security payments, the provision of social and medical help, legal aid and advice, court proceedings, and the emergency services, the cost to the Exchequer must be enormous. Yet the myth persists that somehow matters that are vaguely perceived as domestic and private are really not a social problem and therefore no concern of the State. This myth interferes with people's perception of social reality, fostering an ambivalent attitude often reflected in the unhelpful responses of those called upon for help.

This was well illustrated recently by the experience of a divorcing mother. From her account it will be seen that her desperation increased when faced with a policeman's ambivalence. This, in turn, prompted her to take action which could well have prejudiced her rights to the matrimonial home. Similar ambivalence reflected generally in social policy, and carried to the point where the problem is almost totally denied, can only increase human misery, bringing other social problems in its wake.

> 'I was so frightened of him. Someone had to protect me. He was breaking into the house, you know, in the early hours of the morning, frightening me in bed and things like that. I'd had hospital treatment because of him. I didn't want to leave before because I

was afraid I would lose the house. He had told me so many a time: "If you leave the house it's all mine". I had called the police one night. The policeman said, "Oh well, if he actually kills you, love, or knifes you, we can step in". I said "What am I supposed to do?". There was no-one to turn to, no-one to protect me. That's why I felt I had to leave the house. I was so frightened. The little boy was so upset and in such a hell of a state – you know he was on tablets as well – I just broke down. I just 'phoned my brother at 11 o'clock at night and said "Come and get me as soon as you can". Well, he was there within half an hour. I just packed a few clothes and off I went.'

Notes

1 Some of the current frustrations about the slow pace of law reform and the development of legal services, recently expressed by the Law Society (Lord Chancellor's Office 1982), can be attributed to the same cause.

Appendix

The Practitioner Study: mode of sampling and characteristics of practitioners

Mode of sampling used in the Practitioner Study

In order to obtain comparable samples comprised of fifty practitioners from each of the four occupational groups, the following methods were used.

SOLICITORS

Using the local Law Society's Referral List we approached those firms who undertook family litigation and enquired which staff members specialized in it. We then drew up an alphabetical list of 123 individual solicitors working within a total of seventy-four firms and wrote to every other one. When one refused we substituted the next name on the list. Eighty-three per cent agreed to take part. Most of those who refused had either ceased to specialize in marital work or felt that they could not afford the time.

LOCAL AUTHORITY SOCIAL WORKERS

It proved difficult to obtain a representative sample of local authority social workers. In principle, the Director of Social Services was willing for social workers to take part, but delegated responsibility for the selection to Principal Social Workers. They were told that we wished to interview a representative group of fifty fieldworkers. We were not allowed to select them ourselves from a complete staff list and were given instead a list of fifty 'volunteers'.

HEALTH VISITORS

Our sampling frame was the complete list of health visitors (total 102) working within the old Bristol city boundary. This was provided by

Appendix: The Practitioner Study 209

the Senior Nursing Officer for the Avon Area Health Authority. Since our target was fifty, we wrote to every other one on the list. When one refused we took the next on the list. All but four of those approached agreed to take part.

GENERAL MEDICAL PRACTITIONERS

The sample was drawn from the Avon Family Practitioner Committee's Medical List (1977 edition), comprising 218 doctors working in the Bristol area. Initially we took one in four. When a doctor refused, the next on the list was approached. Fifty-four per cent agreed to take part. In view of the high refusal rate, we wrote to the forty doctors who had declined to ask for their reasons. Twenty-one replied, often with very helpful answers. A number said that they were tired of taking part in research which, as one put it: 'costs the country large sums of money and accomplishes nothing'.[1] Another said: 'the amount of work we do with patients who have problems with marital violence is so small in the context of all the other work we have to do that to spend time actually being interviewed about that minute proportion of our work cannot be justified'. This remark was typical of many. Whatever the reasons, the low response casts some doubt on the representativeness of this sample.

Some characteristics of the practitioners

AGE DISTRIBUTION

There are published national data for social workers,[2] doctors,[3] and lawyers.[4] In the case of health visitors, the Bristol, Southmead, and Frenchay Health Districts supplied us with information concerning all 155 health visitors working in their areas. This gave us some basis for comparison. The age distribution is plotted on Figures 1-4 below. It will be seen that there is a close match between our social workers and the national sample. Our doctors were rather older, 32 per cent falling within the fifty to sixty years old age bracket, compared with 25 per cent for the DHSS survey, and 16 per cent for the National Morbidity Survey (Office of Population Census and Surveys 1979). Our sample of health visitors showed a preponderance in the age range thirty-one to thirty-five.

Comparison between all four samples shows that social workers are, on average, the youngest. The doctors are the oldest, 88 per cent of them being over thirty-six years old, compared with 68 per cent of the health visitors, 34 per cent of the solicitors and 32 per cent of the social workers. The higher average age of the two medical occupational groups is, in part, influenced by the length of their training.

Compared with published data about the age distribution of all practising solicitors (Royal Commission on Legal Services 1979: 52), our sample was, on average, younger. This may be because family litigation in larger firms tends to be taken on by younger, less experienced partners or assistant solicitors.

Figure 1 *Solicitor age distribution*

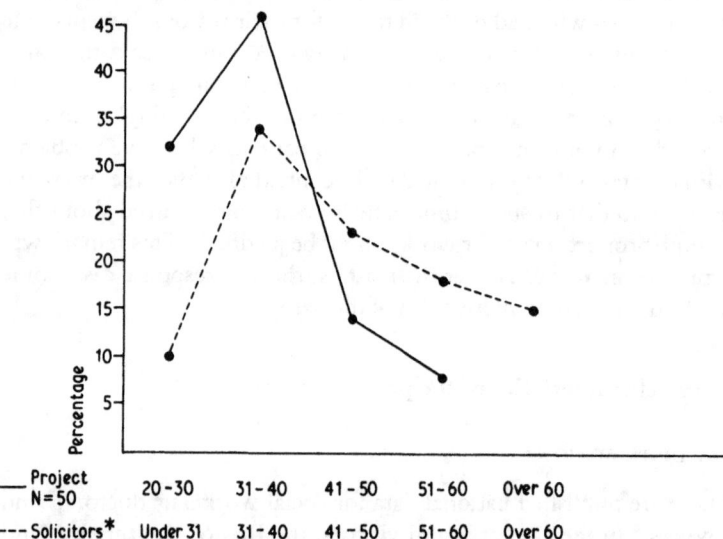

(* Royal Commission on Legal Services, Volume II, Table 1.10. 1979.
N.B: These figures are somewhat misleading because the Royal Commission's data only applied to the 19,247 principals in private practice. There were a further 7,414 assistant solicitors in private practice for whom information about age is not published. They can be assumed to be considerably younger than principals. Our sample might, therefore, be more representative than appears at first sight from this chart.)

Figure 2 *Social worker age distribution*

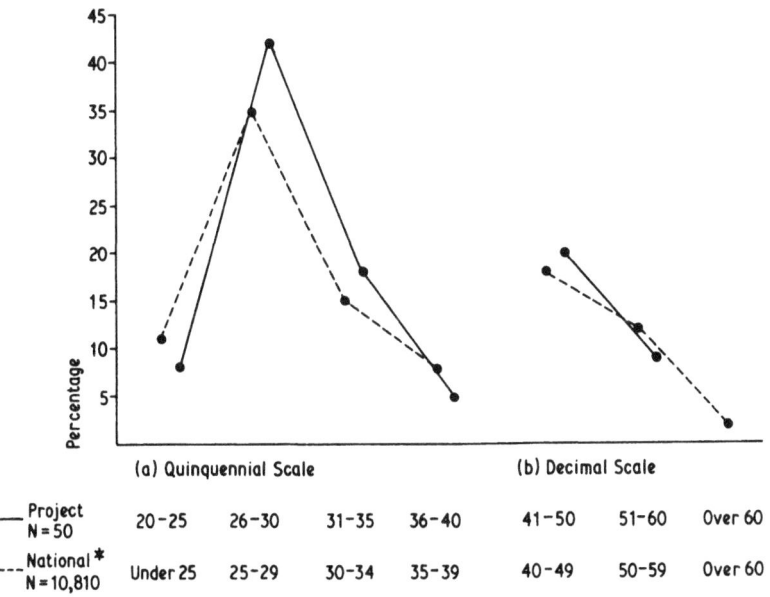

(*Social Workers in Post at 30 September 1977. Figures supplied by DHSS Research Section)

Figure 3 *Health visitor age distribution*

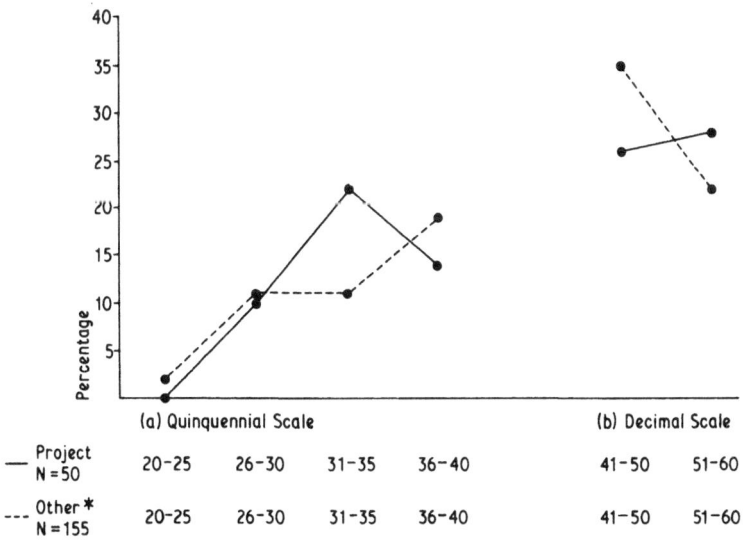

(*Health Visitors in Post in the Bristol, Southmead and Frenchay Health Districts)

Marital Violence

Figure 4 *General medical practitioner age distribution*

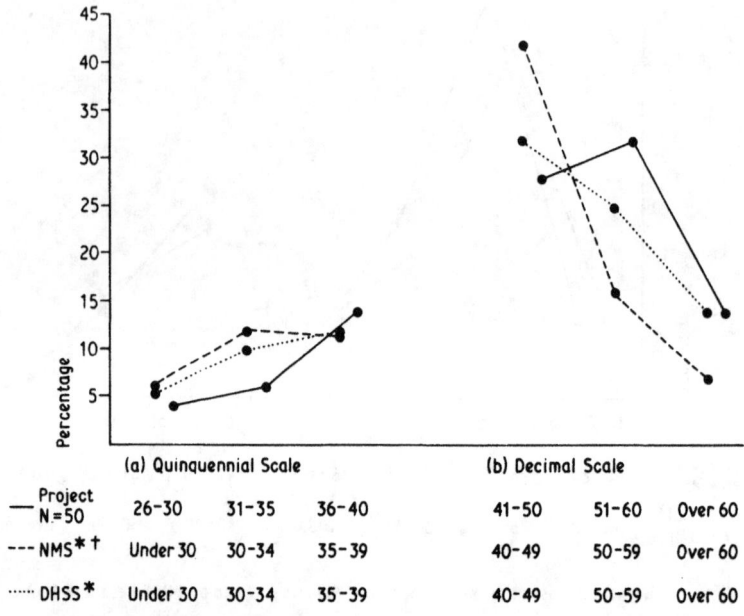

		(a) Quinquennial Scale			(b) Decimal Scale		
——	Project N=50	26-30	31-35	36-40	41-50	51-60	Over 60
---	NMS*†	Under 30	30-34	35-39	40-49	50-59	Over 60
·····	DHSS*	Under 30	30-34	35-39	40-49	50-59	Over 60

(*Morbidity Statistics from general practice 1971-72. Second National Study. Studies on Medical and Population Subjects, No. 3, Table 5.4
† This study was based on data from 43 practices with 60 principal practitioners. See page x and page 1.)

SEX OF PRACTITIONERS

Table 1 *Sex × occupation*

	Solicitors (n = 50) %	Social workers (n = 50) %	Health visitors (n = 50) %	GPs (n = 50) %
M	88	38	–	86
F	12	62	100	14

MARITAL STATUS OF PRACTITIONERS

Table 2 *Marital status × occupation*

	Solicitors (n = 50) %	Social workers (n = 50) %	Health visitors (n = 50) %	GPs (n = 50) %
Married	74	68	46	92
Separated	–	6	–	2
Divorced	–	4	6	–
Cohabiting	–	2	–	–
Widowed	–	–	2	2
Single	26	20	46	4

The doctors and lawyers were predominantly married men. The health visitors were all women, about half of whom were single. Nearly two-thirds of the social workers were female, the majority married.

PROPORTION OF PRACTITIONERS WHO HAVE CHILDREN

The following table indicates the number who were parents.

Table 3 *Parenthood × occupation*

	Solicitors (n = 50) %	Social workers (n = 50) %	Health visitors (n = 50) %	GPs (n = 50) %
No children	44	54	58	6
Children	56	46	42	94

It is clear that social workers and health visitors had the least personal experience of parenthood. It is also notable that the group of doctors predominantly comprised older fathers.

LENGTH OF PROFESSIONAL EXPERIENCE

Practitioners were asked how long they had been practising and how long they had worked in their present practice or area. It should be noted that with the exception of social workers, the length of practitioners' experience was calculated from the time of qualification. Ten social workers were unqualified.

Table 4 *Time spent working in the profession or occupation*

	Solicitors (n = 50) %	Social workers (n = 50) %	Health visitors (n = 50) %	GPs (n = 50) %
Less than 2 years	6	4	4	–
2–5 years	24	44	32	–
6–10 years	38	40	24	14
11–20 years	24	12	24	26
Over 20 years	8	–	14	56
No information	–	–	2	4

These data confirm that the social workers were the least experienced group (48 per cent with less than five years' experience). By contrast, the doctors were the most experienced, although allowance must be made for the fact that they were older. It should also be remembered that after qualifying, doctors spend a number of years working in hospitals before moving into general practice.

Table 5 *Number of years in present practice or area*

	Solicitors (n = 50) %	Social workers (n = 50) %	Health visitors (n = 50) %	GPs (n = 50) %
Less than 2 years	20	46	26	8
2–5 years	36	42	32	12
6–10 years	28	10	22	14
11–20 years	10	2	16	22
Over 20 years	6	–	2	40
No information	–	–	2	4

It will be seen that only six of the fifty social workers had more than six years' experience in their area, compared with corresponding figures of twenty-one health visitors, twenty-two lawyers, and forty

Appendix: The Practitioner Study 215

doctors. Indeed, almost half the social worker sample had worked for less than two years in the area. By contrast, almost half the doctors had been twenty years or more in their practice.

Our impression is that the youngest practitioners in each occupation are the most mobile. This may be particularly true of social workers, many of whom began their careers as unqualified practitioners before training.

Notes

1 A number gave the impression that they had had a surfeit of research which may be a particular problem in a university city with a large Medical School.
2 Data provided by DHSS.
3 See OPCS *National Morbidity Study – Studies on Medical and Population Subjects,* No. 36, 1971-72, Table 5.4, HMSO, 1979, page 24.
4 Report of the Royal Commission on Legal Services, Volume 2, Table 1.10.

References

Abel-Smith, B. and Stevens, R. (1968) *In Search of Justice*. London: Allen Lane.

Abraham, M. (1962) *The Judicial Process*. Oxford: Oxford University Press.

Allen, L. (1978) Child Abuse: A Critical Review of the Research and the Theory. In P. J. Martin (ed.) *Violence and the Family*. New York: Wiley.

Altman, I. (1975) *The Environment and Social Behaviour – Privacy, Personal Space and Territory Crowding*. Monterey, California: Brooks Cole.

Arkell, P. J. (1975) Police Activity Analysis. *Police Research Bulletin* **25**: 8.

Ashley, J. (1973) *Hansard*, 16 July.

Ball, D. W. (1972) Problematics of Responsibility. In J. Douglas (ed.) *Deviance and Respectability – the Social Construction of Moral Meanings*. New York: Basic Books.

Becker, H. (1963) *Outsiders*. Glencoe: Free Press.

Bedfordshire Police (1976) Report on Acts of Violence Committed in the County.

Binney, V., Harkell, G., and Nixon, J. (1981) *Leaving Violent Men. A Study of Refuges and Housing for Battered Women*. Women's Aid Federation.

Boszormenyi-Nagy, I. and Sparkes, G. (1973) *Invisible Loyalties*. New York: Harper & Row.

Byrne, P. S. and Long, B. E. (1976) *Doctors Talking to Patients*. London: HMSO.

Campbell, C. (1976) Perspectives on Violence. In N. Tutt (ed.) *Violence*. London: HMSO.

Chester, R. (1973) Health and Marital Breakdown – Some Implications for Doctors. *Journal of Psycho-Somatic Research* **17**: 317.

Chester, R. and Strether, J. (1972) Cruelty in English Divorce – Some Empirical Findings. *Journal of Marriage and the Family* **34**: 706.

Cobbe, Frances Power (1878) Wife Torture in England. *Contemporary*

Review, April.
Council of the Law Society (1974) *A Guide to the Professional Conduct of Solicitors.* London: HMSO.
Davis, G., Macleod, A., and Murch, M. (1982) Special Procedure in Divorce and the Solicitor's Role. *Family Law* **12**(2): 39.
Denzin, N. K. (1970) Rules of Conduct and the Study of Deviant Behaviour. In J. Douglas (ed.) *Deviance and Respectability – the Social Construction of Moral Meanings.* New York: Basic Books.
Department of Health and Social Security (1979) *Morbidity Statistics from General Practice 1971-72.* London: HMSO.
Derlega, V. and Chiakin, A. (1977) Privacy and Self-disclosure in Social Relationships. *Journal of Social Issues* **33**(3): 102.
Dingwall, R. (1971) *The Social Organization of Health Visitor Training.* London: Croom Helm.
Dobash, R. E. and Dobash, R. P. (1979) Wife Beating – The Negotiation of Daily Life under Patriarchal Domination. Research paper obtainable from the Department of Sociology, University of Stirling.
—— (1980) *Violence Against Wives – A Case Against the Patriarchy.* London: Open Books.
—— (1981) Community Response to Violence Against Wives: Charivari, Abstract Justice and Patriarchy. *Social Problems* **28**(5): 563.
Dobash, R. E., Dobash, R. P., and Cavanagh, K. (1981) Contact Between Battered Women and Service and Medical Agencies. Paper presented to DHSS Conference on Violence in the Family – Recent Research on Services for Battered Women and their Children. University of Kent at Canterbury. September 1981.
Donzelot, J. (1980) *The Policing of Families – Welfare versus the State.* London: Hutchinson.
Elston, E., Fuller, J., and Murch, M. (1975) Judicial Hearings of Undefended Divorce Petitions. *Modern Law Review,* November.
—— (1976) Extract taken from an unpublished research paper, Battered Wives: the Problems of Violence in Marriage as Experienced by a Group of Petitioners in Undefended Divorce Cases. Submitted as evidence to the Parliamentary Select Committee on Violence in Marriage.
Farragher, T. (1981) The Police and Marital Violence. Paper presented at DHSS Seminar on Violence in the Family – Recent Researches on Services for Battered Women and their Children. University of Kent at Canterbury, September 1981.

Franklin, A. W. (1975) *Concerning Child Abuse*. New York: Churchill Livingstone.

Freeman, M. D. A. (1979) *Violence in the Home*. New York: Saxon House.

—— (1980) The Criminal Injuries Compensation Scheme and the Family: A Comment on the Revised Scheme. *Family Law* **10**(2).

Fried, C. (1970) *An Anatomy of Values*. Cambridge, Mass.: Harvard University Press.

Gayford, J. (1978) Battered Wives. In J. P. Martin (ed.) *Violence and the Family*. New York: Wiley.

Gelles, R. J. (1973) *The Violent Home*. Beverly Hills: Sage Publications.

—— (1975) Violence and Pregnancy. *The Family Co-ordinator*.

—— (1978) Violence in the American Family. In J. P. Martin (ed.) *Violence and the Family*. New York: Wiley.

—— (1979) *Family Violence*. Beverly Hills: Sage Publications.

George, V. and Wilding, P. (1972) *Motherless Families*. London: Routledge and Kegan Paul.

Gibson, C. (1974) The Association between Divorce and Social Class in England and Wales. *British Journal of Sociology* **XXV** (1): 79.

Gibson, E. and Klein, S. (1969) *Murder 1957-1968: A Home Office Statistical Division Report on Murder in England and Wales*. London: HMSO.

Goffman, E. (1956) *The Presentation of Self in Everyday Life*. Harmondsworth: Penguin.

—— (1963) *Stigma*. Englewood Cliffs: Prentice Hall.

Goode, W. J. (1971) Force and Violence in the Family. *Journal of Marriage and the Family* **33**(4): 624-36.

Hansard (1976) House of Lords, Vol. 373, Col. 1438.

Haskey, J. (1982) The Proportion of Marriages Ending in Divorce. *Population Trends* **27**. HMSO.

Heider, F. (1958) *Psychology of Interpersonal Relations*. New York: Wiley.

Heisler, J. and Whitehouse, A. (1976) The NMGC Client 1975. *Marriage Guidance* **16**(6): 188.

Homans, G. C. (1961) *Social Behaviour: Its Elementary Forms*. New York: Harcourt, Brace and World.

Home Office Working Party on Marriage Guidance (1979) *Marriage Matters*. London: HMSO.

Ingham, R. (1978) Privacy and Psychology. In J. B. Young (ed.) *Privacy*. New York: Wiley.

Jeffery, L. and Pahl, J. (1979) Battered Women and the Police. Paper given at the 1979 Conference of the British Sociological Association.
Kennedy, I. (1981) *The Unmasking of Medicine*. London: George Allen & Unwin. See also *The Listener*, November and December 1980.
Laing, R. D. (1971) *The Politics of the Family*. London: Tavistock.
Laslett, B. (1973) The Family as a Public and Private Institution: An Historical Perspective. *Journal of Marriage and the Family* **35**(3): 480.
Laslett, P. (ed.) (1972) *Household and Family in Past Time*. Cambridge: Cambridge University Press.
Law Society (1977-78) Report on the Operation of Part 1 of the Legal Aid Act 1974. *28th Legal Aid Annual Reports (1977-78)*. London: HMSO.
Leonard, P. (1981) Lecture given at DHSS seminar on Violence in the Family – Recent Research on Services For Battered Women and their Children. University of Kent at Canterbury, September 1981.
Leonard, P. and McLeod, E. (1980) Marital Violence: Social Construction and Social Service Response. University of Warwick.
Levinger, G. (1966) Sources of Marital Dissatisfaction among Applicants for Divorce. *American Journal of Orthopsychiatry* **XXXVI**: 803.
London Borough of Lambeth (1975) Report of Joint Committee of Enquiry into Non-Accidental Injury to Children, with particular reference to Lisa Godfrey.
Lord Chancellor's Office (1979) *29th Legal Aid Annual Reports*. London: HMSO.
—— (1982) *31st Legal Aid Annual Reports*. London: HMSO.
Marsden, D. (1978) Sociological Perspectives on Family Violence. In J. P. Martin (ed.) *Violence and the Family*. New York: Wiley.
Marsden, D. and Owen, D. (1975) The Jekyll and Hyde Marriages. *New Society* **32**: 333.
Martin J. P. (ed.) (1978) *Violence and the Family*. New York: Wiley.
Mattinson, J. and Sinclair, I. (1979) *Mate and Stalemate – Working with Marital Problems in a Social Services Department*. Oxford: Blackwell.
Matza, D. (1969) *Becoming Deviant*. Englewood Cliffs: Prentice Hall.
May, M. (1978) Violence in the Family – An Historical Perspective. In J. P. Martin (ed.) *Violence and the Family*. New York: Wiley.
McClintock, F. H. (1963) *Crimes of Violence*. New York: St Martin's Press.
MacCormick, D. N. (1974) Privacy: A Problem of Definition. *British Journal of Law and Society* **1**(1): 75.

Miller, D., Pain, D., and Webb, A. (1978) Violence and Conflict in Marriage. Perspectives and Policies. *Social Work Service* **16**: 50.

Miller, N. (1975) *Battered Spouses*. Occasional Papers on Social Administration, No. 57. London: Bell.

Mitchell, A. K. (1981) *Someone to Turn To: Experiences of Help Before Divorce*. Aberdeen: Aberdeen University Press.

Morgan, H. G. (1979) *Death Wishes? The Understanding and Management of Deliberate Self-Harm*. New York: Wiley.

Mortlock, B. (1971) *The Inside of Divorce*. London: Constable.

Moyle, J. B. (1912) *Imperatoris Justininiani Institutiones* (Justinian's Institutes). Fifth Edition. Oxford: Oxford University Press.

Murch, M. (1975) Paper prepared for the Home Office Working Party on Marriage Guidance (Unpublished).

—— (1978) The Role of Solicitors in Divorce Proceedings. *Modern Law Review*, January: 30-7.

—— (1980) *Justice and Welfare in Divorce*. London: Sweet and Maxwell.

Norfolk County Council (1975) Report of the Review Body appointed to enquire into the case of Steven Meurs.

Office of Population Census and Surveys (1979) FM2 No. 3 *Marriage and Divorce Statistics*. London: HMSO.

O'Brien, J. (1971) Violence in Divorce Prone Families. *Journal of Marriage and the Family* **33**: 692–98.

O'Gorman, A. J. (1963) *Lawyers and Matrimonial Cases*. New York: Free Press.

Pahl, J. (1978) *A Refuge for Battered Women*. London: HMSO.

—— (1977) The Canterbury Women's Centre 1975-76. Report available from Centre for Research in the Social Sciences, University of Kent.

—— (1979) The General Practitioner and the Problems of Battered Women. *Journal of Medical Ethics* **5**(3): 117.

—— (1981) A Bridge over Troubled Waters: A Longitudinal Study of Women who Went to a Refuge. Unpublished report for the DHSS.

Parker, S. (1981) The Need for Protection from Violence: The Legal Background. Paper presented at DHSS Seminar on Violence in the Family – Recent Research on Services for Battered Women and their Children, University of Kent at Canterbury.

Parrish, P. A. (1971) The Prescribing of Psychotropic Drugs in General Practice. *Journal of the Royal College of General Practitioners* **21** Supplement 4.

Pizzey, E. (1974) *Scream Quietly or the Neighbours Will Hear*.

Harmondsworth: Penguin.
Reid, W. H. and Schyne, A. W. (1969) *Brief and Extended Casework*. New York: Columbia University Press.
Reisman, J. (1976) Privacy, Intimacy, and Personhood. *Philosophy and Public Affairs*, Volume 6.
Roberts, S. (1979) *Order and Dispute: An Introduction to Legal Anthropology*. Harmondsworth: Penguin.
Royal Commission on Legal Services (1979) *Report: Volume 2*.
Samuels, A. (1978) Privacy: A Legal View. In J. B. Young (ed.) *Privacy*. New York: Wiley.
Scolnick, A. (1973) *The Intimate Environment: Exploring Marriage and the Family*. Boston: Little, Brown.
Scott, R. A. (1970) Construction of Conceptions of Stigma by Professional Experts. In J. Douglas (ed.) *Deviance and Responsibility: The Social Constructions of Moral Meanings*. New York: Basic Books.
Select Committee on Violence in Marriage (1975) *First Report*. London: HMSO.
Society of Conservative Lawyers (1981) *The Future of Marriage*. London: Conservative Political Centre.
Somerset Area Review Committee for Non-Accidental Injury to Children (1977) *Wayne Brewer: Report of the Review Panel*. Somerset County Council.
Steimetz, S. K. and Straus, M. (1974) *Violence in the Family*. New York: Harper & Row.
Straus, M. A. (1977) Wife Beating: How Common and Why? In Eekelaar and Katz (eds) *Family Violence*. London: Butterworth.
Thomson, J. J. (1975) The Right to Privacy. *Philosophy and Public Affairs* 4(4): 295.
Tracey, R. (1974) *Battered Wives*. A report by the Bow Group. London: Bow Publications.
Walster, E., Walster, G. W., and Berschied, E. (1978) *Equity Theory and Research*. Boston: Allyn & Bacon.
Wasoff, F. (1981) Violence to Women in the Home: A Research Strategy. Paper presented at DHSS seminar on Violence in the Family – Recent Research on Services for Battered Women and their Children. University of Kent at Canterbury, September 1981.
Westcott, J. (1977) Family Problems: The Solicitor and his Client. *Family Law:* 7(1) 24-9.
Westin, A. (1967) *Privacy and Freedom*. New York: Atheneum; London: The Bodley Head (1970).
Wilson, E. (1976) *The Existing Research into Battered Women*.

National Women's Aid Federation.
Winkler, J. T. (1981) The Political Economy of Administrative Discretion. In M. Adler and S. Asquith (eds) *Discretion and Welfare*. London: Heinemann.
Women's Aid Federation in England (1981) Violence to Women in the Home: A Research Strategy.
Younger (1972) Report of the Committee on Privacy. Cmnd 5012. London: HMSO.

Name Index

Abel-Smith, B., 138
Abraham, M., 141
Allen, Letitia, 28–9
Altman, I., 109
Arkell, P. J., 21
Ashley, Jack, 7, 11
Avon and Somerset Constabulary, 18, 21

Ball, D. W., 78
Baker, Sir George, 95
Becker, H., 79
Bedford Police, 11
Berscheid, E., 184
Binney, V., 28, 29, 30, 34, 185, 189
Boszormenyi-Nagy, I., 184
Bristol Royal Infirmary, 16
Byrne, P. S., 187

Campbell, C., 43
Cavanagh, K., 167
Chester, R., 4, 166 fn., 186
Chiakin, A. 109
Cobbe, Francis Power, 3
Community Response to Marital Violence, Bristol Project, 3
Council of the Law Society, 103, 135, 144, 165 fn.

Davies, Jean, 82, 83
Davis, G., 29 fn., 191
Dawson, Barbara, 10
Denzin, N. K., 78–9
Department of the Environment, 80 fn., 134 fn.
Department of Health and Social Security, 4, 134 fn.

Derlega, V., 109
Dingwall, R., 152, 153
Dobash, R. E., 27, 30, 36, 52, 56, 60 fn., 79–80, 111, 124, 159, 167, 185, 188, 191, 192, 202–03
Dobash, R. P., 27, 30, 36, 52, 56, 60 fn., 79–80, 111, 124, 159, 167, 185, 188, 191, 192, 202–03
Donzelot, J., 202
Dow, Chief Superintendent, 115, 193

Elston, E., 5, 65

Farragher, Tony, 10, 29 fn., 134 fn., 193
Finer Committee, 191
Frankenburg, Professor R., 10
Franklin, A. W., 82, 83
Freeman, M. D. A., 52, 134 fn.
Fried, C., 108
Fuller, J., 5, 65

Gayford, J., 56
Gelles, R. J., 28, 41, 52, 56, 65, 113
George, V., 190
Gibson, C., 35
Gibson, E., 28
Goffman, E., 78, 111
Goode, W. J., 56, 109
Guardian, The, 204

Hansard, 7, 128–29
Harkell, G., 28, 29, 30, 34, 185, 189
Haskey, J., 27
Heider, F., 12
Heisler, J. 15
Homans, G. C., 184

Home Office Working Party on Marriage Guidance (1979), 135, 159, 160, 165 fn., 168, 188, 189, 198 fn.

Ingham, R., 107, 108
Inter-Departmental Committee on Conciliation, 191

Jeffery, L., 134 fn., 192, 195

Kennedy, I., 60, 77
Keyte, Chief Superintendent, 193
Klein, S., 28

Laing, R. D., 76
Laslett, B., 112, 113
Laslett, P., 112
Legal Action Group, 134
Leonard, P., 56, 203
Levinger, G., 26–7
London Borough of Lambeth, 4
Long, B. E., 187
Lord Chancellor's Office, 116, 117
Lyon, Alex, 3

McClintock, F. H., 28
MacCormick, D. N., 97
McLeod, E., 56, 203
Macleod, A., 29 fn., 191
Marsden, D., 53, 55, 65, 73, 77
Martin, J. P., 95
Mattison, J., 147, 165 fn., 167, 190
Matza, D., 78
May, M., 3, 56, 75
Miller, D., 55
Miller, N., 11, 41, 167
Mitchell, A. K., 166 fn., 186, 190, 191
Morgan, H. G., 193–94
Mortlock, B., 135, 140
Moyle, J. B., 184
Murch, M., 5, 35, 65, 114 fn., 135, 144, 166 fn., 184, 186, 190, 191, 196

National Women's Aid Federation, 4–5, 31, 65
Nixon, J., 28, 29, 30, 34, 185, 189
Norfolk County Council, 4

O'Brien, J., 4, 56
Office of Population Census and Surveys, 31, 209, 215 fn.
O'Gorman, A. J., 136
Owen, D., 65

Pahl, J., 10 fn., 31, 116, 134 fn., 159, 185, 186, 187, 190, 192, 195
Pain, D., 55
Parker, S., 128
Parrish, P. A., 64
Phillips, Baroness, 128–29
Pizzey, Erin, 4, 56, 201

Reid, W. J., 166 fn.
Reisman, J., 108
Roberts, Simon, 184
Rowntree, Joseph, Memorial Trust, 29 fn.
Royal College of General Practitioners, 159, 187
Royal Commission on Legal Services, 210, 215 fn.

Samuels, A., 113 fn.
Scott, R. A., 78
Select Committee on Violence in the Family, 4
Select Committee on Violence in Marriage, 3, 4, 8, 11, 52, 115, 127, 168, 193, 201, 206
Shearer, Ann, 204
Shyne, A. W., 166 fn.
Sinclair, I., 147, 165 fn., 167, 190
Skolnick, A., 77
Society of Conservative Lawyers, 202
Somerset County Council, 4
Southmead Hospital, 16
Sparkes, G., 184
Steimetz, S. K., 28, 52

Stevens, R., 138
Straus, M., 28, 42, 52
Strether, J., 4

Thomson, J. J., 108
Times, The, 3
Times Law Report, 95
Tracey, R., 4

Walster, E., 184
Walster, G. W., 184

Wasoff, F., 134 fn.
Webb, A., 55
Welsh Office, the, 134 fn.
Westin, A., 109
Westcott, J., 135
Whitehouse, A., 15
Wilding, P., 190
Wilson, E., 5
Winkler, J. T., 199–200
Women's Aid Federation, 204

Younger Committee, 97

Subject Index

Age: practitioners, 149–50, 170, 177–78, 190, 209; victims, 31–2
Agencies: clients' needs, 183–84, 185, 197; help-seeking from, 185–96; use and referral, 35–7, 111, 159, 185, 189, 190
Alcohol and violence, 14, 55, 56, 57, 60, 61, 75, 203
Ambivalence: practitioners, 115, 118, 123, 125, 206; in social policy, 206
Ambivalent clients, and general medical practitioners, 186, 187; health visitors, 118; police, 115–16, 117; social workers, 116, 118–19; solicitors, 93, 116
Avon Council on Alcoholism, 37 fn.; number of marital violence cases noted, 14–15, 18
Avon Family Practitioner Committee's Medical List, 209
Avon and Somerset Constabulary, 18, 21

Boundaries and frontiers of services, 178
Bristol Women's Aid, 22, 37, 116, 130; numbers referred to refuge, 22–3

Case studies, 65–75
Child saving, 90, 201, 204, 205
Children, and confidentiality, 102–05, 106; non-accidental injury to, 4, 28, 82–8, 94–5; of 'marital' partnership, 33–4; at risk, 89, 95; and social workers, 150–51
Chiswick Women's Aid Refuge, 4, 201

Citizens' Advice Bureau, 37 fn., 200; number of marital violence cases noted, 15, 18, 130
Cohabitation, length of, 33
Collaboration between services, 168, 189, 197–98, 198 fn.
Conciliation, inter-departmental committee on, 191; services, 191–92, 200
Confidentiality, 97, 102–07; and children, 102–05, 106; general medical practitioners, 102–03, 105–07, 160, 186, 187; health visitors, 102–03, 105–06; primary health care team, 105–07; social workers, 102–03, 105–06; solicitors, 103–04; *see also* Privacy
Court: divorce, 4, 7, 25, 26; family, 191, 200
Court proceedings, 195–96, 200
Criminal Injuries Compensation Scheme, 127

Data collection problems, 12–13
Definition of marital violence, 8, 13; criteria, 43–7; discussion, 50–1; form of, 42–3; method of approach, 41–2; views about, 47–50
Department of Health and Social Security, 3, 9, 187, 189, 191, 201, 204–05; Homelessness and Addictions Research Liaison Group, 4, 204
Deviance, 73, 74, 78, 79–80 fn.
Dispute, fair treatment in, 184
Divorce, 5, 25, 26, 27, 35, 80 fn., 128–29, 191, 206; *see also*

Subject index 227

Injunctions
Divorce court, 4, 7, 25, 26; solicitors' duty to, 143, 165 fn.
Divorce court welfare officers, 196
Divorce Reform Act 1969, 5
Divorce research, 5, 26, 29 fn., 111, 114 fn., 158, 184, 186
Divorcing parents, 158–59
Doctors, *see* General Medical Practitioners
Domestic Violence and Matrimonial Proceedings Act 1976, 10 fn., 125, 128; *see also* Injunctions
Domiciliary Statutory Social and Medical Services, 17–18, 126; *see also* Health visitors; Social workers
Drugs, medically prescribed, and marital violence, 63–4
Emergency Legal Aid Certificates, 195
Emergency services, 192–94; medical, 192–93; police, 193–94; refuges, 194–95; voluntary specialist, 139

Evidence: discussion, 94–5; marital violence, 88–94; non-accidental injury to children, 82–8; *see also* Proving marital violence
Experience, practitioners' length of, 214–15
Explanation of marital violence: case study illustrations, 65–72; discussion, 75–9; medical, 62–5, 75; method of approach, 54–5; method of classification, 55–7; quantitative data, 57–65

Familism, 201–02, 204, 205
Feminism, 56, 202–03, 204, 205

General Household Survey, 24
General Medical Practitioners, 9, 30, 35, 37 fn.; and ambivalence, 186–87; case studies, 71–2; characteristics of, 209, 210, 212–15; and children of marital violence, 163, 164; and client withdrawal, 119, 120, 121, 122, 123; and confidentiality, 102–03, 105–07, 160, 186, 187; consultation with, 6, 24–5, 158, 186; counsellor and friend, 161; definition of marital violence, 43, 44, 45, 46, 47–51; explanation of marital violence, 59, 60, 61, 62–4, 71–2, 74; help-seeking from, 186–88; knowledge of the law, 132–33; and non-accidental injury to children, 86–8; number of marital violence cases noted, 23–5; and other partner of marital violence, 163, 164–65; and privacy, 91, 101–02; and proof of marital violence, 90–1; restricted to medical help, 160, 162–63, 172, 187; and retrenchment policy, 200, 205; role definition, 156–65; sampling mode, 209; scope of responsibility, 163–65; use of, 36, 158–59, 183; viewed by other services, 152, 172, 177
Green Form Scheme, 137, 165 fn., 191, 195; *see also* Legal Aid and Advice Scheme

Health visitors, 9, 30, 36; and ambivalence, 118; case studies, 69–71; characteristics of, 209, 210, 212–15; and children, 172; client withdrawal, 120, 121; and confidentiality, 102–03, 105–06; definition of marital violence, 43, 44, 45, 47–51; explanation of marital violence, 59, 60, 61, 62–4, 69–71, 74; knowledge of the law, 129–31; liaising with doctors, 86–7, 88, 152, 171; liaising with other services, 153, 154–55, 169, 171, 177, 178, 187–88; as marital counsellor, 155; neutral stance, 156; and non-accidental injury to children, 17, 82–5; number of marital violence cases noted, 17, 18; partisan role of, 155–57; and privacy, 97–101; and proof of marital violence, 88–90; role definition, 151–57; sampling mode, 208–09; scope of responsibility, 155–57; social welfare role, 153, 154; supportive listener, 153; viewed by other services, 152, 170–72, 177, 178

Help-seeking, in early stages of marriage breakdown, 183, 186–90; at termination of marriage, 183, 190–92; *see also* specific practitioner

Hospital accident departments, 30, 193, 194; marital violence cases noted by, 16, 18

Housing (Homeless Persons) Act 1977, 110, 129, 134 fn.

Ideological conflict, 203–04

Injunctions, 6, 7, 10 fn., 25, 26, 91, 92, 93, 96 fn., 117, 118, 125, 128, 132, 133, 137, 138, 191, 193, 195

Law: civil, 128–29; criminal, 126–28; practitioners' understanding of, 126, 129–34

Lawyers, *see* Solicitors

Legal aid, 117, 191; and retrenchment policy, 200

Legal Aid Act 1974, 165 fn.

Legal Aid and Advice Scheme, 137, 138, 165 fn.; *see also* Green Form Scheme

Liaison between agencies, 86, 94, 193; *see also* Collaboration

Liaison officer (CPV), 85, 86

Local Authority Social Services, 7, 34, 85, 88, 110, 131, 134, fn., 139, 147, 148, 158, 165 fn., 169, 170, 171, 194; help-seeking from, 189–90

Local Authority Social Workers, *see* Social workers

Marital status of practitioners, 177–78, 213

Marital violence: definition, 8, 13, 42 ff.; discussion, 26–9; evidence of, 5, 7, 12, 21, 25, 26, 28, 88–94; explanation of, 52 ff.; locality variations, 19; number of cases, 11, 14–27, 206; and privacy, 12, 81–2, 97 ff.; and proof, 88–94; prosecutions for, 19–21; social characteristics of victim, 26–7; *see also* Victim

Marriage, length of, 27, 33

Marriage Guidance Council, 15, 31, 111, 148, 149, 157, 161, 162, 167, 171, 190, 193, 200; Bristol, 15, 30; Catholic Marriage Advisory Council, 15, 30; help-seeking from, 188–89; marital violence cases noted by, 15, 18; use of, 36; viewed by other services, 172–75, 178–79

Marxism, 203

Matrimonial Causes Act 1878, 3; 1973, 25, 110

Matrimonial Proceedings Magistrate's Courts Act 1978, 10 fn., 128

Medical explanations for violence, 62–5, 75

Medical services in emergency, 193–94

National Morbidity Survey, 23, 24, 25

National Society for the Prevention of Cruelty to Children, 84, 86, 103, 104

Neutral stance, 184, 185, 189; *see also* specific practitioner

Offences Against the Person Act 1861, 21, 127

Partisanship, 100, 184, 185, 189; of health workers, 156–57; social workers, 149–50; solicitors, 100,

Subject index 229

135–36, 139–41, 169
Personality and violence, 55, 56–7, 60–1, 75
Police: and ambivalence, 115–16, 117, 206; Avon and Somerset Constabulary, 18, 21; emergency service, 192–93; help-seeking from, 192–93; intervention, 7, 21–2, 81, 110, 111, 127, 133, 161, 186, 192–93, 206–07; marital violence cases noted, 18–22; neutrality, 192; prosecutions for marital violence, 19–21, 127, 186, 195–96; and retrenchment policy, 200; study of marital violence cases, 11; use of, 36, 130
Policy considerations: ideological conflict, 203–04; reformist ideologies, 201–03; retrenchment, 199–201, 205; social justice, 205–07
Poverty and violence, 55, 60, 75
Practitioners, *see also* specific practitioner; characteristics of, 209–15; client choice of, 196–97; parental status of, 213–14; sampling mode, 208–09; study of, 9–10, 208 ff.; views of each other's services, 167–79
Pregnancy and violence, 64–5
Primary health care team, 152, 153, 189, 194, 198; and confidentiality, 105–07
Privacy, 12, 97–102, 185, 186; and influence on public awareness of marital violence, 111–12; and intimacy in personal relationships, 108–09; nature of, 107–110; and neighbours, 84–5, 86, 88, 89, 90, 95; and possible increase of marital violence, 112–13; *see also* Confidentiality
Probation, 103, 133, 196
Probation Service, 133
Proving marital violence: general medical practitioners, 90–1; health visitors, 88–90; independent witnesses, 93; medical evidence, 93–4; mutual allegations, 93; police, 127; social workers, 88–90; solicitors, 91–4
Proving non-accidental injury to children: general medical practitioners, 86–8; health visitors, 82–5; social workers, 85–6

Referral to other services/agencies, 36–7, 107, 167
Reformist ideologies, 201–03
Refuges, 4, 5, 7, 22–3, 27, 29, 31, 34, 37, 110, 111, 124, 132, 159, 168, 175–77, 194–95, 200, 202–03; Bristol, 22–3, 116; Canterbury, 31, 185; Chiswick, 4, 201; funding of, 194–95, 205; viewed by other services, 175–77
Research, Community Response to Marital Violence, 3; background, 3–4; method of approach, 13–15; objectives of 7–8; feasibility study, 8–9, 97, 129, 136, 144
Research, general: need for, 4–5; and retrenchment policy, 200, 205; previous, 5–7
Research Projects: Bristol Divorce Research, 55, 158, 184, 186; Circumstances of Families in Divorce Proceedings, 111, 114 fn.; Sheffield NWAF, 65; Special Procedure in Divorce, 26, 29 fn.
Role definition: general medical practitioners, 157–65; health visitors, 151–57; social workers, 147–51; solicitors, 135–47

Samaritans and confidentiality, 111
Select Committee on Violence in Marriage, 3, 4, 8, 11, 52, 115, 127, 168, 193, 201, 206
Sex of practitioners, 213, 177–78
Social justice, 205–07
Social workers, 7, 9, 30; and

ambivalent clients, 116, 118–19; case studies, 67–9; characteristics of, 209–11, 213–15; and child interviewing, 150–51; and client withdrawal, 117, 118, 119, 120, 121, 123; and confidentiality, 102–03, 105–06; definition of marital violence, 43, 45, 46, 47–51; explanation of marital violence, 58, 60, 61, 67–9, 74; as family therapists, 151; help-seeking from, 190; knowledge of the law, 129–30, 131–32; liaison with doctors, 87; and male partner of marital violence, 149–50; marital violence cases noted, 18; neutral stance, 149; and non-accidental injury to children, 18, 85–6, 112; partisan role of, 49–50, 191; and privacy, 97–101; and proof of marital violence, 88–90; role definition, 147–51; sampling mode, 208; use of, 36; viewed by other services, 169–70, 177, 178, 190

Solicitors, 7, 9, 30, 35, 183; and ambivalent clients, 93, 116; case studies, 65–7; characteristics of, 209, 210, 211–15; and children, 140, 141, 142, 143, 144, 146–47; and confidentiality, 103–04; counselling role of, 136, 137–38; definition of marital violence, 42, 43, 44, 45, 46, 47–51; diagnoser of problems, 137; duty to the court, 143, 165 fn.; emotional involvement, 140; explanation of marital violence, 58, 60, 61, 65–7, 74; help-seeking from 190–91; marital violence case estimates, 25–6; neutral stance, 139, 140, 141; and other family members, 141, 142–47; partisan role of, 135–36, 139–41, 144, 169; and privacy, 98, 99, 100; and proof of marital violence, 91–4; role definition, 135–47; sampling mode, 208; scope of role, 141–43; social work role, 138; use of, 36; viewed by other services, 168–69, 177; welfare rights adviser, 138–39

Stigma, 6, 11, 78, 95, 111, 121, 158, 168, 171, 186, 190, 191, 197, 204; see also Deviance

Stress and violence, 55, 56, 60, 62, 159, 160, 201

Symptoms of marital problems, 160, 162

Victim of marital violence, 12, 24, 42, 44, 78, 126, 128, 159; age, 24, 31–2; children of partnership, 33–4; length of marriage/cohabitation, 33; personality, 7, 60–1, 79; sex, 31; socio-economic status, 7, 26–7, 29, 34–5

Vignette test, 130–32

Violence: and alcohol, see Alcohol; and children, see Children; medical explanation for, 62–5, 75; and personality, 55, 56–7, 60–1, 75, 192; and poverty, 55, 60, 75; and pregnancy, 64–5; and stress, 55, 56, 60, 62, 159, 160, 201

Violent men, 3, 5–6, 27, 41, 42, 51 fn., 52, 78, 81, 92, 93, 109, 156, 167, 188, 192, 195–96, 202–03, 206–07

Violent women, 28, 42, 51 fn., 52, 93

Voluntary specialist services, 14–16, 139, 193; see also specific service

Withdrawal by client, 116; discussion, 123–25; health visitors' response to, 118; social workers' response to, 118–19; solicitors' response to, 117–18

Withdrawal, reasons for, 119–23, 124

Women's Aid Federation, 4, 13, 167, 200, 204; and confidentiality, 111

Women's Aid Groups, 127; as viewed by other services, 175–77, 178; see also Refuges